CHANGING PATTERNS
IN PSYCHIATRIC CARE

CHANGING PATTERNS
IN
PSYCHIATRIC CARE

An Anthology of Evolving Scientific

Psychiatry in Medicine

COMPILED AND EDITED BY

THEODORE ROTHMAN, M. D., F. A. C. P.

University of Southern California
School of Medicine, Los Angeles

Rush Research Foundation
LOS ANGELES, CALIFORNIA
AND
Crown Publishers, Inc.
NEW YORK
1970

Printed in the United States of America
Published simultaneously in Canada by
General Publishing Company Limited

TYPOGRAPHY BY TERE LO PRETE

This volume is dedicated to Dr. Paul H. Hoch, investigator, teacher, administrator, who not only left his inspired mark upon the leadership of the American College of Neuropsychopharmacology, and upon so many of its members, but who also embraced intellectually almost all the fields represented in the spectrum of the reports that comprise this volume

Contents

PERSPECTIVES IN THE ETIOLOGY AND TREATMENT OF AFFECTIVE DISORDERS

NEW APPROACHES TO RESEARCH AND EDUCATION

CHANGING PERSPECTIVES
IN PSYCHIATRIC CARE

Acknowledgments

I wish to thank the Board of Directors of the Rush Research Foundation for their encouragement and support in the publication of this volume. The Foundation and I are most grateful to the first Sustaining Members of the Rush Research Foundation, Inez and Donald Rubendall, La Canada, California, whose generous financial sponsorship helped so greatly to make this volume possible. Previous gifts by these dedicated friends also have supported several new investigations.

Thanks are due Mrs. Jo Hawkins, whose unswerving dedication and devotion to the American College of Neuropsychopharmacology and as Associate Director of the Foundation lent inspiration to all as she worked constantly at my side during the assembling and editing of this work. Deep appreciation goes to Dr. Milton Greenblatt, Commissioner of Mental Hygiene, the Commonwealth of Massachusetts, for his suggestions, for his gentle encouragement, and for his advice emanating from a depth of scientific wisdom and experience.

I also wish to thank the distinguished Fellows and Members of the American College of Neuropsychopharmacology, together with their scientific co-workers and friends, whose unique symposia and studies constitute the chapters—the very backbone—of this book. Gratitude is expressed, too, to the Writers Consultation Service, UCLA Extension, which provided the services of Walter R. Schmidt as editorial assistant; and to my wife, Jean, for her patience and forebearance during those many trying hours when my preoccupation with the manuscripts that comprise this volume became a virtual obsession.

T.R.

Contributors

WILLIAM S. APPLETON, M.D.

Instructor of Psychiatry
  Harvard Medical School
Director of Clinical Psychopharma-
  cology
  Massachusetts   Mental   Health
    Center
  Boston, Massachusetts

CHING-PIAO CHIEN, M.D.

Assistant Clinical Professor of Psy-
  chiatry
  Tufts Medical School
Director, Southwest Boston Mental
  Health Center
  Boston State Hospital
  Boston, Massachusetts

JONATHAN O. COLE, M.D., F.A.P.A.

Superintendent
  Boston State Hospital
  The Commonwealth of Massa-
    chusetts
  Department of Mental Hygiene
Professor of Psychiatry
  Tufts University School of Medi-
    cine
  Boston, Massachusetts

JOHN M. DAVIS, M.D.

Chief, Unit of Clinical Pharma-
  cology
  Laboratory of Clinical Science
  National   Institute   of   Mental
    Health
  Bethesda, Maryland

ALBERTO DiMASCIO, PH.D.

Director of Psychopharmacology
  for the State of Massachusetts
Associate Professor of Psychiatry in
  Psychopharmacology
  Tufts Medical School
  Boston, Massachusetts

JEAN ENDICOTT, PH.D.

Senior Research Scientist
  Washington Heights Community
    Service
  New York State Psychiatric Insti-
    tute
  Biometrics   Research,   New   York
    State
  Department of Mental Hygiene
    and
  Columbia University, Depart-
    ment of Psychiatry
  New York, New York

DAVID M. ENGELHARDT, M.D.,
  F.A.P.A.

Professor of Psychiatry
  State University of New York
  Downstate Medical Center
  Brooklyn, New York

MAX FINK, M.D., F.A.P.A.

Professor of Psychiatry and Director
  Division of Biological Psychiatry
  New York Medical College
  New York City

KURT GORWITZ, SC.D.

Director of Mental Health Statistics
Maryland Department of Mental
Hygiene
Director of the Maryland Psychiatric
Case Register
Baltimore, Maryland

MILTON GREENBLATT, M.D., F.A.P.A.

Commissioner, Massachusetts De-
partment of Mental Health
Professor of Psychiatry
Tufts University School of Medi-
cine
Boston, Massachusetts

TURAN M. ITIL, M.D.

Professor of Psychiatry and
Associate Chairman
Department of Psychiatry
University of Missouri School of
Medicine
St. Louis, Missouri

ALI KESKINER, M.D.

Assistant Professor of Psychiatry
University of Missouri School of
Medicine
St. Louis, Missouri

DONALD F. KLEIN, M.D., F.A.P.A.

Director of Research
Hillside Hospital
Glen Oaks, New York

SIDNEY LEVENSTEIN, D.S.W.

Research Associate
Hillside Hospital
Glen Oaks, New York

REUBEN A. MARGOLIS, PH.D.

Assistant Professor of Psychiatry
State University of New York
Downstate Medical Center
Brooklyn, New York

PHILIP R. A. MAY, M.D., F.A.P.A.

Clinical Director, Neuropsychiatric
Institute
State of California Department of
Mental Hygiene
University of California
Los Angeles
Clinical Professor of Psychiatry
University of California at Los
Angeles, School of Medicine
Los Angeles, California

ALVIN M. MESNIKOFF, M.D.

Director, Washington Heights Com-
munity Service
Associate Clinical Professor of Psy-
chiatry
Columbia College of Physicians
and Surgeons
Professor of Psychiatry
State University of New York
Downstate Medical Center
Director, South Beach Psychiatric
Center
Staten Island, New York

ROBERT F. PRIEN, PH.D.

Research Psychologist
Central Neuropsychiatric Re-
search Laboratory
Veterans Administration Hospital
Perry Point, Maryland

BERNARD ROSEN, M.A.

Staff Psychologist
Hillside Hospital
Glen Oaks, New York

THEODORE ROTHMAN, M.D., F.A.C.P.,
F.A.P.A.

Clinical Professor of Psychiatry
University of Southern California
School of Medicine
Attending Psychiatrist, Los Angeles
County-University of Southern
California Medical Center
Executive Director
Rush Research Foundation
Los Angeles, California

RICHARD I. SHADER, M.D.

Assistant Professor of Psychiatry
Harvard Medical School
Director of the Psychopharmacology
Research Laboratory
Associate Clinical Director, and
Principal Psychiatrist
Massachusetts Mental Health
Center
Boston, Massachusetts

SIROON P. SHAHINIAN, PH.D.

Research Associate
Hillside Hospital
Glen Oaks, New York

MYRON R. SHARAF, PH.D.

Director of Sociopsychological Re-
search and Training
Boston State Hospital
Assistant Clinical Professor of Psy-
chiatry (Psychology)
Tufts University School of Medi-
cine
Boston, Massachusetts

JOVAN SIMEON, M.D.

Assistant Professor of Psychiatry
New York Medical College
New York, New York

ROBERT L. SPITZER, M.D.

Director, Research Division
Washington Heights Community
Service
New York State Psychiatric Insti-
tute
Biometrics Research
New York State Department of
Mental Hygiene
Department of Psychiatry
Columbia University
New York, New York

GARFIELD TOURNEY, M.D., F.A.P.A.

Professor of Psychiatry
University of Iowa
College of Medicine
Iowa City, Iowa

Preface

The rapid changes and shifting emphases in psychiatric thought have spanned so relatively brief a time that even within my professional career of less than three decades I have witnessed the multitudinous concepts and resultant programs that comprise the dynamic era of today's psychiatry.

In 1941, when I first ventured upon the wards of a mental hospital, psychiatry was déclassé among the medical specialties; physicians generally considered it a hopeless field. Mental hospitals were custodial warehouses. The prevailing intellectual emphases were on classification of disease, the minutiae of elaborate case histories, and scholarly references to Bleuler and Kraepelin. Psychoanalysis was enthusiastically supported by a handful of men, influenced often by a trip to Vienna or personal contact with Freud. In our medical schools, medicine and surgery dominated the field. Psychiatry as a discipline was poorly regarded since its beliefs and practices were considered as lacking adequate scientific foundation. Only the mediocre medical student, or the extremely curious, gravitated toward a career in our field.

The beginning of change was evident by 1941. Shock therapy, insulin therapy, and lobotomy became major concerns in the education of psychiatric residents. As a result of these techniques there was witnessed dramatic improvements and/or recovery in patients formerly classified as hopeless or destined for lengthy hospitalization. Also, as residency programs began to take formal shape, the teaching of psychotherapy as a separate modality and the supervision method of instruction became central features of postgraduate education. A serious study of psychodynamics became part of the background necessary for close communication with patients. It became customary to search deeply into patients' feelings, thoughts, and communications, with the therapist doggedly learning to spend countless hours remaining "cool" while a patient revealed the contents of his primitive, archaic unconscious.

By the late 1940s—certainly by the 1950s—psychoanalysis and psychotherapy had won the field and, because of their fascination, had permeated every branch of behavioral science. No sooner had these assumed an apparent secure place in the psychiatric firmament, however, than a new dimension began to gain recognition—namely, social (and later, community) psychiatry.

It has been stated that just as the rise of psychoanalysis dominated the first half of the 20th century, so will the evolution of social and community psychiatry dominate the second half of the 20th century. Yet this simple formulation must also be modified to embrace the "somatic recrudescence" resulting from new pharmaceuticals and the widening interests in psychopharmacology. In many ways, the present scene has developed into one more complex and more eclectic than in any previous period of our history.

While these trends were being established, major socio-political shifts began to irreversibly alter the psychiatric picture through the rapid assumption of responsibility by local, state, and especially national governments for the welfare of the health, including the mental health, of the public. This constitutes one of the most heartening and effective developments of our recent past, the involvement of the body politic effecting a consequent rising tide of identification by the public with the cause of mental illness and retardation. State and federal governments have poured many millions into research, demonstration, construction, staffing, and into fostering new programs such as comprehensive community mental health centers, total health multiservice centers, partnership with the people, model cities, and also into the beginnings of epidemiology and preventive psychiatry. Individual citizens and citizen groups by the many thousands have volunteered their services to mental health and retardation facilities; in many states, these volunteers have assumed responsibility for part of—and in some instances all—the mental health developments in their neighborhood.

Another interesting feature—and a critically important one—that has characterized the changing times is to be observed in the growing significance of research and the research point of view in psychiatry. In the early 1940s psychiatric research was woefully weak, limited as it was largely to laboratory investigations, clinical classifications or frequently esoteric applications of classic psychologic laboratory techniques to diagnosis or prognosis. The science of methodology was a virtual myth; rigorous application of experimental design or of statistical validation was just beginning to surface, and the use of behavioral scales was in a primitive stage of development. At that time very few of the young men and women who entered psychiatry possessed the skill, the training, or the financial backing to pursue a problem in a scientific style, no less pursue it over a period of years. Our field lagged greatly behind the swiftly advancing fields of medicine and surgery; we paid a considerable price in self-esteem for these shortcomings as compared to the esteem enjoyed by our nonpsychiatric colleagues.

Time has brought change. In all levels of concern—psychologic, sociologic, biologic—new researchers have been trained, supported, and given tenure to generate programs of research of a sort that would stand the scrutiny of very critical specialists. Today the impact of their contributions is being effectively realized. There has been very salutary emphasis on design, on sophisticated analytic techniques, and on long-term follow-through. More and more of our young scientists have become able to speak an interdisciplinary language, or at least can collaborate fruitfully with the variety of specialists in behavioral science who together are striving to comprehend man, well or sick, in his infinite complexity.

This was indeed the early setting in which men such as Joel Elkes, Paul Hoch, Theodore Rothman (the editor of this book), and others with similar interdisciplinary interests foregathered in 1960 to organize the American College of Neuropsychopharmacology (ACNP). Viewed in the light of the present, the ACNP is a society of elite scientists whose studies in psychopharmacology are actually vigorous collaborations in concert with a multitude of other specialists. The college gives appropriate significance to interdisciplinary efforts and offers a forum from which any one discipline is prepared to speak to all the others. In our earlier psychiatric scene this was unusual, almost unique. ACNP workshops have instigated a variety of books and symposia in an attempt to offer the latest word on the multidisciplinary approaches at those respectable levels of scholarship and understanding that lend credence to the subjects reported upon.

Under Dr. Rothman's editorship, selected new research contributions stimulated chiefly by the ACNP have been brought together to give the reader a discriminating view of the changing face of psychiatry as presented by those working and shaping their new field.

Milton Greenblatt

President, American College of
  Neuropsychopharmacology (1964)

Commissioner of Mental Health,
  Commonwealth of Massachusetts

Introduction

"The truth is that medicine professedly founded on observation, is as sensitive to outside influences, political, religious, philosophic, imaginative, as is the barometer to atmospheric density."*

The historian, Crane Brinton, once predicted to me that our contemporary sexual revolution would eventually evolve into a new puritanism. The historian frequently sees social and political movements as transient phenomena that soon are modified by rendering definitions to accepted phrases, thus changing the original meaning and direction or, with time, causing the movement perhaps to shift to an opposite direction. Schopenhauer believed that social movements are similar to a pendulum swinging to the left and right. Ideas are kaleidoscopic images.

Concepts that influence the lives of men have the transience of mankind itself. Yesterday's self-evident convictions are today's waning beliefs. Psychiatric therapeutic movements change like women's fashions. Each of these movements has charismatic leaders and worshiping followers who uncritically practice their beliefs; convinced of omnipotence, they influence psychiatric thought for a number of decades, then give way to other leaders who develop their own personality cults. Most of the resulting beliefs are closer to religious fervor than science.

T. H. Huxley maintains that "science commits suicide when it adopts a creed." Sciolism very often takes the place of science and metaphors the place of scientific experiments. One case in point is the controversial history of phrenology. Precipitated onto the stage of the 18th and 19th centuries through its founder, Franz Joseph Gall (1758–1828), the theory and treatment played a significant role in medicine, philosophy, and literature. Phrenology was spread throughout the European scientific, cultural, and intellectual world by Gall's disciples. In 1832 Johann Casper Spurzheim (1763–1832), a disciple, came to lecture in the United States. He died in Boston within a few months and was given a hero's burial. Whereupon the *American Journal of Medical Science* lamented, "The prophet is

* Holmes, Oliver Wendell: *Medical Essays: Currents and Counter Currents in Medical Science.*

gone, but his mantle is upon us." When George Combe, another Gall disciple, arrived in America, he too was acclaimed by the outstanding intellectuals. Medical men, including many psychiatrists, as well as political, cultural, and literary leaders—among them Horace Mann, Walt Whitman, Edgar Allan Poe, and President James Garfield—were most enthusiastic about this sciolism.

Phrenology, following the history of other sciolisms, waxed and waned as a social movement. With the advent of scientific neurology, phrenology was reduced to a footnote in the history of ideas.

Psychiatric ideas that bridged the gap from 18th- and 19th-century speculative fashions to our 20th-century popular convictions began with Franz Anton Mesmer (1734–1815). Mesmer was a Viennese physician who began in the 1770s to obtain dramatically successful individual and group results with a method he called "animal magnetism," popularly called "Mesmerism." Mesmer's belief was that the universe was filled with a magnetic fluid, and man's health depended upon its amounts and its distribution. Cures were achieved by a laying on of hands by a magnetist. In Paris, in 1778, he attracted a considerable following. He also was creating enemies and was exposed to the most violent accusations of charlatanism. In 1784, after being rebuffed by a Royal Commission of Louis XVI made up of Lavoisier, Bailly, Benjamin Franklin, and Dr. Guillotine, he retired from public life to Bodensee, Switzerland.

Though it was easy to refute Mesmer's simplistic beliefs in magnetism, his extensive therapeutic successes impressed many practical clinicians. As a result, Mesmerism as a practice spread widely throughout France, Germany, Great Britain, and the United States. In America, Mary Baker Eddy practiced as a Mesmerist and later founded the Christian Science religion. Mesmerism passed through many phases, refining its theories and practices. The clinical experiences were called Neurohypnology by James Braid (1795–1860). James Esdaile (1808–1859) did numerous surgical procedures under what now began to be called hypnosis, and many other surgeons followed.

The foremost physician of his time, Charcot, viewed hypnosis as an interesting clinical experience, and demonstrated it at Salpetrière. A general practitioner, A. A. Liebeault from Nancy, France, believed this clinical experience was therapeutic and concluded that the major factor was suggestion. Hippolyte Marie Bernheim, professor of medicine at Nancy, championed Liebeault's belief that suggestion could be used for psychologic healing. Young physicians such as Forel and Freud came to Nancy to study these methods of suggestion. Many clinical experiments now were studied by such renowned experimentalists as Charles Richet and Rudolf Heidenain, and were practiced by such outstanding psychiatrists as Freud, Bleuler, Moebius, and others.

A wave of reaction against hypnosis and suggestion began in the late part of the 19th century. Ottomar Rosenbach employed "rational" waking psychotherapy. In 1900 Paul Dubois was joined by Dejerine in treating patients with moral therapy called persuasion. Pierre Janet began studying early traumatic memories in the hypnotic state and the way these memories could cripple early development. Morton Prince and A. Binet elaborated this cathartic method and studied multiple personalities.

Sigmund Freud was among the most celebrated physicians of the early 20th century, his name ranking with the foremost physicians of history. He molded the psychiatric ideas that had emanated from France into his own personal ideology, which became an international movement. Ideas have their ecology, and the early part of the 20th century enthusiastically gathered Freud's psychology, metapsychology, and philosophy and created a body of knowledge that became one of the fervent speculative convictions of our era.

During the past 50 years, psychoanalysis has had an enormous impact on American psychiatry, medicine, art, literature, child rearing, philosophy, social sciences, and all the media of expression: cinema, television, radio, newspapers, and magazines. Today, psychoanalysis is besieged by a crescendo of criticism from some of its leaders. Szasz says: "Psychoanalysis is vanishing. It is as moribund and irrelevant as the Liberal party in England."* Marmor warns: "Psychoanalysis is in danger of receding into an unimportant sidestream of psychiatry." Freud's metaphoric language brought him closer to being an ally of poetry than of the scientific method. Thornton Wilder reports that Freud told him: "The poets have always sensed what psychoanalysis has discovered." Bettelheim calls Freud's psychoanalysis "time-bound, very shaky, very dubious." Phelps believes that the further we become removed from Freud, the more his truth seems like a personal, poetic vision rather than an impersonal, scientific investigation.† A disquieting survey

---

* Most of the quotations in this Introduction are from "Crossroads in Psychoanalysis," by Leo, Frank: *The New York Times,* 8/4/68. p. 1.

† Phelps, Robert, *Twentieth-Century Culture: The Breaking Up,* Introduction, New York: George Braziller, 1965, p. 271.

made recently by the National Institute of Mental Health noted that of 40 recognized forms of psychiatric therapy used in the United States, only 2% received psychoanalytic therapy, and this percentage is rapidly decreasing.

As federal funds and the mental health centers expand, briefer and more easily administered therapies are being used. Psychoanalysis never prepared itself to fulfill the urgent and current needs of the new community psychiatry. Psychoanalysis reached its zenith in the 1950s, and the fervor of its adherents continues to wane. It failed to keep pace with other current psychiatric multidisciplinary approaches. Redlich was disturbed in the 1960s that "almost everything we know about psychoanalysis was Freud's single-handed and single-minded." Harold Kaplan and Redlich see the psychoanalytic world as a rigidly dogmatic and defensive guild, stagnant and unprepared by its rigidity to find creative solutions to current problems. Kelman reports a gradual loss in the number of psychiatrists applying to the psychoanalytic institutes for training, from one out of seven in 1945 to one out of twenty today.

The true failure of psychoanalysis is that, unlike other medical sciences, it has not evolved sufficient scientific research programs. Engel, writing in the *Journal of the American Psychoanalytic Association,* sadly notes: "The failure of psychoanalysis to mount productive research programs during 15 years of generous support from the National Institute of Mental Health and foundations, is heading for a general reappraisal by granting agencies of their policy and support. Much of the blame will have to be laid at the doors of those who have failed to recognize the obligation to develop research psychoanalytic scientists as well as practitioners."

Redlich angrily charges that "psychoanalysts are systematically excluding candidates with creative minds. Analysts, particularly those in the Association, have created a tightly controlled shop through a careful system of educational supervision and control. One could almost speak of censorship. The boundaries are tight. There is little room for the doubter, the critic, the maverick."

Psychoanalysis' great contribution to psychiatry is its emphasis on a dynamic frame of reference. It helped shape to a large extent our thinking and intellectual currents. It did enrich psychiatry with the invaluable psychodynamic approach.

At present, new social and political creeds are in ferment; the problems of urbanization, overpopulation, the crises of youth, and the care of the masses of people from all social strata are on stage demanding our attention. Our current scientific and social climate is in need of a new type of psychiatrist and psychiatry with new frames of reference; he must be skeptical, better trained in medicine and research; flexible and creative; he must prepare himself to accept the complex challenges of today's problems by using the new evolving multidisciplinary approaches relevant to our time and to our new research methods in psychiatry.

Psychopharmacology is the bridge from the psychiatric beliefs of the mid-20th century that propelled psychiatry to undergo its long-delayed scientific revolution and brought it forward to become a medical science. Psychopharmacology has helped produce a binding of the multidisciplinary approaches to psychiatry in medicine involving the social, biologic, and psychologic with the use of experimental designs where variables can be measured, which in turn has evolved use of sophisticated biostatistics and programming.

The main purpose of this book is to inform the reader concerning some of the changing directions of psychiatric care in medicine. Its chapters elucidate the sophisticated social, clinical, and scientific methods now being widely used by multidisciplinary research teams to help obtain new tentative findings. The emphasis throughout this volume is to avoid firm convictions, magic slogans, and to offer scientific flexibility to clinicians, research teams, and teachers. Speculation, though encouraged, is considered rational guessing and is held not as truth but as a means to explore new hypotheses to be tested by well-designed experiments.

The moral conviction of this volume follows the spirit of the American College of Neuropsychopharmacology (ACNP): it is better to admit ignorance than to be a blind believer; it is better to observe and test in the clinic and laboratory than write polemics concerning one's own metaphors; it is better to be skeptical and tentative in one's beliefs than have untestable, firmly held speculations. Many of the authors are members of the ACNP or are associated with ACNP Study Groups.

This volume is divided into six sections that elaborate on changing patterns of psychiatric care. No attempt is made to present all the changes; however, a small number have been chosen to support and illustrate the ACNP thesis, illuminating significantly new clinical research and educational trends. Reporting, as they do, carefully devised research methods and supporting scientific conclusions, some of the chapters will challenge our readers, thus instigating a heated but illuminating silent cerebral dialogue.

The plan of our sections is pyramidal. The first section is the foundation, the historic background of psychiatric therapies—their rise and fall. The second section builds on this foundation with a series of contributions of current "happenings" in psychiatric care, delineating the mental hospital in transition, the programming of new community mental health and walk-in services. The contribution of biostatistic data, gathered in the Maryland Psychiatric Case Register, and its use in determining the changing patterns of psychiatric care are also reported. The pyramid continues upward with the third section, which contains a series of controlled studies on the treatment of schizophrenia, varying from the most effective community care therapies to hospital treatments. Presented also are special chapters on minimizing drug use and prolonging drug holidays; the effectiveness of the use of large doses of chlorpromazine; and the bimonthly intramuscular use of fluphenazine. Section Four offers a detailed study on the newer perspectives of affective disorders; the etiology of affective disorders and the biogenic amine hypothesis are reviewed. The variety of modalities for treatment of manic-depressive states and their subtypes is surveyed. The implications for clinical practice, future research, and psychiatric education are suggested. The fifth section reports a miscellaneous group of perspectives involving the problems in research and psychiatric education, plus a presentation of a variety of pragmatic suggestions helpful to investigators and educators. The search for a unitary psychopathology is studied and shown to be unproven. The final chapter in this section suggests extensive reforms in psychiatric education. The concluding section of the book is a critical appraisal of psychiatric care, representing a summary and discussion of this work.

The chapters that comprise this volume,* written by challenging investigators, are certain to stimulate the reader. Some chapters may evoke anger, some are sure to be criticized, and others perhaps will delight a few. Whichever the effect, this book exposes the reader to a newer type of research man. Start it with a flexible mind and it can help reformulate some of your firmest convictions—convictions that quite possibly need to be reformulated, to meet the changing patterns in psychiatric care.

Theodore Rothman, M.D.
Editor

* The editor's comments appear in italics at the beginning of each chapter.

HISTORIC EVOLUTION
OF PSYCHIATRIC CARE

1

*Psychiatric Therapies: 1800–1968**

by GARFIELD TOURNEY

The contemporary psychiatrist must study the history of psychiatric ideas. With the frequent innovations being introduced into psychiatry, a need is created for better frames of reference so that a new label is not mistaken for a new idea, and social movements for advances in therapy. Tourney relates in this chapter how current enthusiastic and highly accredited therapies often lose their appeal after a brief initial trial.

This is an old story. The history of medicine has always been involved in a dialectic struggle between the magic expectations compounded from novel speculations and empiric scientific beliefs. The intellectual milieu has influenced the medical and psychiatric theories prevalent for many centuries. Scientific observation has coexisted with magic speculation. Rational and irrational ideas have lived side by side with ideal humanitarian moral approaches and sadistic inhuman practices.

Tourney shows that it is the charismatic leaders of psychiatry who create ideologies, which predominate and then wane after a brief ascendancy. Our present psychiatric expectancies and anticipations, he points out, have never been so optimistically high, but there is warning that we have had similar historic periods that have waxed and waned. No Cassandra, Tourney enlightens us so that we can view the hope in the new approaches while discriminating their scientific value. Enthusiasm must be proportionately linked with good science. The skepticism is humane, moral, and evinces wisdom. His warnings encourage us to be more skeptical and less influenced by the fashions of therapeutic movements in psychiatry. His conclusion is optimistic as he points out that

* This chapter is a completely revised and enlarged version of a paper that appeared in the *American Journal of Psychiatry,* Vol. 124, 1967, reproduced by permission of the American Psychiatric Association.

new scientific directions are being investigated by a small group of be-
*havioral scientists who are leading us to a hopeful future.**

INTRODUCTION

In 1792 Pinel broke the chains of the insane at Bicêtre and brought
to fruition the humanitarian tradition in psychiatry, an optimistic
and forthright approach to the mentally ill that proved to be a
rational system of therapeutics. Pinel reacted to medical dogmatists
with their strict formalism, rigid doctrines, traditional therapies,
and speculative systems, by seeking the basis for his teachings in
everyday clinical problems. He followed the empirical viewpoint
that through personal observation and humane attitudes a practical
therapy could be developed; he thus revolutionized the care of the
insane. Pinel stated, "Let not the results of experience and observation be compounded with the errors of a doctrine depending for its
support upon prejudices, hypotheses, pedantry, ignorance, and the
authority of celebrated names."[1]

At the beginning of the 19th century, the treatment of the
mentally ill, according to Pinel, consisted of a "curious compound of
pharmacy, superstition and castigation." Hellebore since ancient
times had been regarded as a specific, and many other compounds
were recommended that had passed from one generation to another
for hundreds of years. Emetics, purgatives, and bleeding represented techniques deeply rooted in the humoral theory. The biases
of sin, possession, and witchcraft, relative to insanity, were seen in
primitive measures that included flagellation, seclusion in dark
fetters, the production of fright, and many contrivances for
mechanical restraint. Realizing the antitherapeutic nature of these
approaches and their hypothetic basis, Pinel, in his humane approach, rejected restraints and avoided all cruel treatment of the
insane. He emphasized the need for occupational activities, permitted a limited degree of liberty, and, finally, attached little importance to the use of drugs. Concerned about the natural course of
insanity, he believed that through reliance on nature many cures
could be achieved. "I then discovered that insanity was curable, in

* The remarks in italics preceding the various chapters are Dr. Rothman's editorial
comments.

many instances, by mildness of treatment and attention to the state of the mind exclusively, and when coercion was indispensable, that it might be very effectually applied without corporal indignity."

A similar empiric approach was made by the English Quaker philanthropists, William, Henry, and Samuel Tuke, representing three generations of hospital reformers in England. The major principle of care at their institution, the Retreat at York established in 1796, was that of a humane kindness to patients and a freeing of the insane from neglect, maltreatment, chains, and starvation. In Samuel Tuke's *The Description of the Retreat*, published in 1813, there is a rejection of the medical treatment of the day, with due emphasis placed upon moral treatment that "comprehends all those means which, by operating on the feelings and habits, exert a salutary influence, and tend to restore them to a sound and natural state."[2] The treatment consisted of confinement in a hospital with pleasant surroundings, a general promotion of the patients' comfort, hygienic measures, adequate diet, occupational and educational activities, a limited degree of personal freedom, and the use of coercion and restraint only when deemed absolutely necessary. Positive rather than negative aspects of the functioning of the insane were stressed, such as the patients' degree of self-control.

It is apparent that in these reforms and therapeutic measures are embodied many of the fundamental goals we continue to seek today in the care of the mentally ill. The importance of the historical perspective in relationship to the development, application, and results of therapeutic procedures from 1800 to the present is delineated by a waxing and waning of interests with a frequent defining of needs; it is a history of reports of many new discoveries and treatments, of overoptimism in therapy, followed by pessimism, and of psychiatrists' establishing therapeutic movements that attracted followers. Many so-called specific treatment measures were introduced, only to be forgotten in a brief span of time. Though surgical, mechanical, medicinal, and psychotherapeutic approaches have been described by the thousands, the statement made by Esquirol in 1838 regarding psychiatric treatment still rings true: "It will often be necessary to vary, combine and modify the means employed; for there is no specific treatment of insanity. As this malady is not identical in every case; as in every instance it depends upon the different causes, and presents varied characteristics, and requires new combinations, [there is] a new problem to be solved for every patient whom we are called to treat."[3]

Admittedly, effective treatment measures were developed, including thyroid extract for myxedema madness, niacin for the dementia of pellagra, and penicillin for the treatment of general paresis. On the basis of understanding causal mechanisms and their modification through such treatments, preventative measures were established for these three disorders. The history and conquest of general paresis remains a paradigm of etiologic and therapeutic triumph in the field of psychiatry that has both stimulated and hindered subsequent psychiatric developments.

Many psychiatric disorders may not fit into the model of general paresis. Likewise, other claims of efficacy for specific psychiatric treatment measures have been assumed, such as psychoanalysis as a specific psychotherapeutic technique for the psychoneuroses, insulin coma in schizophrenia, and convulsive therapy in the depressions. Today the efficacy of psychoanalysis has been frequently questioned by psychoanalysts themselves, with many investigators feeling that it has no advantage over psychotherapies based on other theoretic models. The efficacy of insulin therapy has been doubted for years, and it is rarely used now, having been superseded by the tranquilizing agents. Antidepressive medication is rapidly replacing much of the use of electroconvulsive treatment (ECT) for depressions, although ECT continues to have an important place in the therapeutic armamentarium.

As one views the development of psychiatric therapies since the time of Pinel, he is impressed by the life cycle of new treatment methods. The initial enthusiasm and the report of remarkable results today are tempered by the application of more critical study and evaluation, resulting in less impressive statistics. When a method is accepted it is with many limitations, or it is rejected as being of questionable or negligible value. Initial statistics often indicate results of 90% recovery or marked improvement, whereas subsequent studies find these figures reduced to 50%–60% in psychoneuroses, and to 30%–40% in schizophrenia. Often such therapeutic developments become more like a religious movement, strongly identified with a particular leader—observed in psychoanalysis with Freud or insulin therapy with Sakel—than a scientific development. Rejected techniques are often reintroduced in new guises with new names and new theoretic foundations. This type of circular movement has been observed in the application of moral therapy, hospital treatment, psychotherapy, and drug and physical therapies. Too often psychiatric treatment reflects some of the social and political philosophies of the day, rather than a sound medical orientation applying the scientific laws of cause and effect.

Within the past decade, with a tempering of the initial enthusiasm that accompanied the introduction of the tranquilizers, there has been increasing concern regarding research methodology in the evaluation of psychiatric therapies, particularly the various psychopharmacologic agents. More objective techniques are being developed for the measurement of behavior and physiologic processes in responses to drugs. The importance of an interdisciplinary approach by the clinician and basic scientist has been readily acknowledged. As the neurologic bases of behavior become better understood, as well as the dependence of drug response on its situational and social setting, specific therapeutic measures may be discovered for a number of puzzling psychiatric disorders.

Our current approaches conceivably could lead to specific treatment methods analogous to those that first led to the conquest of general paresis, myxedema, and pellagra.

MENTAL HOSPITAL DEVELOPMENTS

What impact did this revolutionary approach to the care of the mentally ill have during the early 19th century? Perhaps the most important of all was an attitude of optimistic enthusiasm developed in the treatment of the mentally ill. Through hospitalization of the insane, the organization of mental hospitals and their specialized personnel, and the application of moral and humanitarian treatments, remarkable therapeutic strides were made. The application of statistical methods to psychiatry as introduced by Pinel also became widespread, and led to the compilation of a great collection of data to help prove the curability of insanity. Some results of treatment at Bethlem Hospital prior to the time of the hospital reform have been reported by Haslam.[4] Many exaggerated claims were made for the private madhouses that existed in England during the 18th century. Francis Willis, who attended George III during his first mental illness, claimed that he could cure nine out of ten patients.[5] Asylums began to report regularly the results of their treatment. In 1849 Isaac Ray wrote: "No subject connected with insanity possesses so deep and general an interest as its curability, and this fact has led to the universal practice among asylums of reporting the number of their recoveries."[6]

TABLE 1

Results of Psychiatric Hospital Treatment

	Date	Re-covered Im-proved	Un-improved & Died	Total	% Recovered & Improved
Bethlem (Haslam)	1784–94	574	1,090	1,664	35
Salpetrière (Pinel)	1803–07	473	529	1,002	47
Retreat (Tuke)	1796–1811	72	77	149	48
Salpetrière (Esquirol)	1804–14	1,218	787	2,005	61
Burrows, Recent Cases	1820	222	20	242	92
Hartford Retreat (Hall)	1827	21	2	23	91
Bloomingdale (Earle)	1821–44	1,094	747	1,841	59
Worcester (Woodward)	1839–43	448	474	922	49
US Asylums	1844	857	1,235	2,092	41
US Asylums	1859	2,576	1,897	4,473	57
Worcester	1880–84	264	1,055	1,319	20
New York State (May)	1912	1,610	5,628	7,238	22

The results of psychiatric hospital treatment from the late 18th century into the 20th are summarized in Table 1. The limitation in the presentation of such data is readily admitted, since the methodologies of reporting statistics vary among individuals and at various periods of time; also, patient populations are by no means comparable, criteria for cure and marked improvement vary, and follow-up data is infrequently presented. However, the Table 1 statistics express important therapeutic attitudes, from optimism to nihilism. Statistics can be manipulated in many ways to promote programs to the medical profession, the general public, and to government officials; hence biases are introduced into any reporting of statistics.

Pinel reported an increase in therapeutic effectiveness as revealed in his early study,[1] as did a later revelation by Esquirol.[3] According to Table 1, for the years 1784 to 1794 at Bethlem Hospital, Haslam listed the cure rate at 35%; Pinel's early study at Salpetrière was 47%, and Esquirol's study reached 61%. Tuke reported a cure rate of 48%.[2] These studies included both acute and chronic patients. Even more impressive are the results as illustrated in Burrows' private practice, where he claimed 92% cures for recent cases,[7] and the small sample of cases from the Hartford Retreat of 91% cures.[8]

These later statistics were reported by Captain Basil Hall, an Englishman, who wrote of his personal travels in America and emphasized that the American civilization had greatly contributed to the cure of the mentally ill in contrast to the limited therapeutic results in England. His statements were frequently quoted in periodicals and newspapers, and on the basis of this remarkably small number of cases, a movement Deutsch[9] called the cult of curability was established. It was generally accepted, as Kirkbride stated, that 80% to 90% of recent cases could be cured.[10]

The therapeutic principles employed by the above-named psychiatrists are admirable in many ways, and form the foundation for a number of our treatment programs today. As Butler stated,[11] patients were to be approached with "courage, kindness, and patience." The secret of moral therapy was believed to rest in kindness and in occupation; the therapeutic dictum was that *the insane should never be idle*. Occupation through labor on the farm and in workshops, education, physical activity, recreational programs, use of confidential and private interviews, emphasis on self-control, proper diet, rest, and the discreet use of drugs characterized the care of patients. A psychologic attitude on the part of the physician was regarded as important, and the role of the childhood experience, as well as moral factors, in the precipitation of illness was recognized. Programs were aimed at the promotion and stimulation of healthy thought. Hospitals should remain small, no more than 250 beds, with the superintendent maintaining personal contact with his patients. A model institution following these principles of therapy was the State Lunatic Asylum at Worcester, established in 1832 under the direction of Samuel W. Woodward. For the years 1834–1843, in his annual reports Dr. Woodward reported a curability rate between 82% and 91.5%.[12] He was able to present such a report through an interesting manipulation of statistics frequently used at that time. The percentage of cures was based on the number of discharges, not admissions; patients who remained in the hospital or who died during the course of their illness were disregarded. However, Dr. Woodward also reported his cures in relationship to total admissions, as presented in Table 1, showing the rate of cure for the years 1839–1843 as 49%.

Conolly advocated a system of total nonrestraint in 1839.[13] Though the use of restraint had been greatly reduced by following the precepts of Pinel and Tuke, many alienists believed in the therapeutic nature of restraint. This became an issue strongly debated in the psychiatric literature printed in the United States from the 1850s to the 1880s. The issue can in many ways be attributed to the continued influence of Benjamin Rush upon psychiatry in this country. Regarded as the father of American psychiatry, Rush was a dogmatist in his approach to mental illness, his theories emphasizing that madness was primarily a manifestation of "morbid excitement in the blood vessels of the brain."[14] His therapy was traditional, and on the basis of his theory of the hyperemia of the cerebral vessels, he strongly advocated bleeding. He devised many complicated means of restraint, which he called tranquilizers. He advocated emetics, purges, blisters, terror, solitude, darkness, cold douches, and other primitive measures in the treatment of the insane. Rush gave no indication of his therapeutic results, which it can be presumed were not impressive.

The Retreat into Custodialism

Results from the mental hospitals throughout the country were compiled and printed collectively until 1860. Table 1 shows that 41% of patients were reported cured or markedly improved in 1844,[15] and as many as 57% in 1859.[16] Subsequently, a gradual decline in therapeutic effectiveness occurred; by 1880 there was a retreat into custodialism and a breakdown of moral therapy. For the five-year period from 1880 to 1884, the cure rate at the Worcester State Lunatic Asylum was reduced to 20% of admissions as compared with 49% forty years previously.[17] Pliny Earle, in 1876, had published his first study titled *The Curability of Insanity,* in which he carefully reviewed the statistical material, including the original reports of Burrows, Hall, and Woodward. He pointed out that in a period of 30 to 40 years a constantly diminishing number of recoveries were reported. Statistics for 30 institutions during their first five years of operation as compared with their last five years of operation revealed that recoveries decreased from 46% to 34%. Earle concluded that recoveries were increased by reporting the repeated recoveries of the same person. On this basis, it is impossible to ascertain from most statistical reports the actual number of persons who recovered. He also pointed out that the number of reported recoveries were influenced largely by the temperament of the reporter, each man having his own criteria for insanity and its cure. Statistical manipulation of figures occurred by basing the percentage of recoveries on patients discharged rather than patients admitted. In any case, the initial patient samples were too small to lend validity. More extensive experience has discredited the assumed curability of insanity as made by the early alienists.

Earle quotes Isaac Ray, who in 1844 stated that "he would be a bold man who should venture to say that Pinel and Esquirol, whose medical treatment was confined chiefly to baths and simple bitter drinks, were less successful in their cure of mental diseases than those numerous practitioners who have exhausted upon them all the resources of the healing art." Earle then concludes:

> If the assertion was true 32 years ago, it is believed that the contents of this exposition sufficiently prove that it is, to say the least, nonetheless true at the present day. The years of a generation have passed since that time, and, in the course of their progress, remedy after remedy before untried has come up big with the word of promise to the hope, but essentially breaking it to experience. Hashish was experimentally tried, proved a failure, and is now nearly forgotten. Chloroform and ether have become convenient and useful to a certain extent, but they have no curative power previously unknown in other remedies. Electro-magnetism, upon which great hopes were placed, is very beneficial in a few cases of disordered nervous action, but hitherto has proved itself powerless to correct those functions the abnormal operations of which constitute insanity.

These attitudes toward the curability of insanity as stated by Earle dominated the attitudes of most hospital psychiatrists until the introduction of the insulin and convulsive therapies in the 1930s. The attitudes excepted, of course, the developments in the understanding of the etiology and treatment for general paresis, myxedema, and nutritional deficiencies with psychosis. Was Pliny Earle correct in his assessment of the situation? Did he take into account other factors—social, cultural, psychologic, and medical as well as statistical—which influenced the reporting of therapeutic results? It must be remembered that in his younger days Pliny Earle, then an enthusiastic therapist, reported a cure rate of 59% at the Bloomingdale Asylum for the years 1821–1844.[18] Earle also utilized biased statistical manipulation in order to increase his own recovery rate, thereby decreasing his own validity, as noted by Bockoven.[19]

Many factors led to the change in attitude that finally culminated in Earle's work relative to the curability of insanity. One of these was a change in psychiatric leadership, the early moral therapists being succeeded by men who viewed insanity as being strictly a cerebral disease. Dr. John P. Gray, who became superintendent at the Utica State Hospital in New York in 1854 and editor of the *American Journal of Insanity* in 1855, posts he held for 30 years, strongly interpreted mental disorder according to disordered cerebral pathology. He rejected the earlier alienists' views that moral factors or passions—ie, emotions—precipitated insanity, and "rightly" proved through his statistics that the immediate causes of insanity were physical.[20] He also supported the use of restraint as having therapeutic value in some instances.

The rapid growth in hospital size proved to have a deleterious effect on patient care. The early psychiatrists had small hospitals. Kirkbride, for example, felt that no hospital should have more than 250 beds.[21] Population growth, immigration with its admission of many of the foreign poor, led to larger and larger hospitals. The proportion of chronic patient admissions was fostered through Dorothea Dix's efforts; many patients previously cared for in charity houses, country homes, and by their own families were now being hospitalized. On admission, patients were—often too readily—classified as curable. Many debates occurred at professional meetings and in the literature as to whether curables and incurables should be treated together or separated in various hospital units.[22] Hospital superintendents were overwhelmed with administrative responsibilities, and lost personal contact with their patients. Thus was established a pattern of hospital administration that remains characteristic for most present-day hospital superintendents. By the 1870s a large number of hospitals had patient populations of over a thousand. Such increments have continued until the present time. Until 1856 the Association of Medical Superintendents defended 250 beds as the maximum size for a state hospital. But the pressure for larger institutions could not be resisted. New York built a 600-bed institution at Utica. The American Association of Hospital Superintendents then defended a 600-bed policy. Later, New York built the Willard State Hospital with 1,500 beds. A recommendation of a ceiling structure of 1,500 beds has never been maintained.[23] Personnel problems, budgetary difficulties, hospital overcrowding, the large proportion of chronic cases, and a dogmatic depersonalized theoretic orientation to insanity led to the growing therapeutic nihilism. Psychiatrists spoke of an increase in both the incidence and severity of illness, which seemed to indicate that civilization was proving to be too much for man.[24] The great achievements of the early moral therapy and the early hospital development were forgotten, to be renewed generally only within the past 20 years.

During the same time, many of the basic principles of modern hospital care and community organization have been emphasized and to some extent realized. Patient treatment was individualized, and open-door policies, permissiveness, and patient freedom were encouraged.[25] Voluntary admissions were advocated as a general procedure by Allen in 1837.[26] Ellis, who spoke of the hospital as a community, established a program of aftercare and arranged employment for his patients.[27] Seymour was a strong advocate, in the 1840s, of home and aftercare.[28] In many cases, only short periods of hospitalization were deemed necessary, with many patients being treated by a general physician in the patients' own homes. He was strongly in favor of systematic visitation to patients by friends and relatives, rather than patient isolation. Furthermore, Seymour believed that most patients could be returned to their homes or family-care units even if not fully recovered. Most of his concepts are similar to current approaches believed to be new therapeutic discoveries.

In 1859 Arlidge[29] emphasized that a gigantic asylum is a gigantic evil, the general management is unwieldy, and due medical and moral care and supervision an impossibility. Staffs are inadequate, personnel are charged with duties that can never be performed, and personal contacts with patients are impossible. The patient's individuality is lost as he becomes a member of a machine with precise regularity and invariable routine—not an apparatus calculated to restore his pristine condition and his independent self-governing existence. Gaskell[30] a year later stressed the need for immediate treatment centers for acute and mild cases in units comparable to our current general hospital units.

However, the pessimistic attitude persisted. Hospitals became more isolated from the general medical community, and often hospital management could be clearly characterized as inhumane and neglectful.[31] Thus a decline began in the last quarter of the 19th century, which continued into the 20th. May's statistical studies showed a decline in recovery rated to 22% in 1912.[32] Budgetary difficulties and lack of personnel led to few changes in the system for a number of years. Recoveries and discharge rates had declined to below 10% in many institutions by the 1920s. Many psychiatrists believed that less than 5% of schizophrenic patients could be expected to recover. Deterioration in patient care and patient improvement undoubtedly reflected the attitudes of the psychiatrists. Deterioration and incurability became linked together. Bleuler's concept that no patient was ever to be considered hopeless was all but ignored. He intimated that much of the pathologic behavior of patients resulted from their hospital experience, rather than their mental illness.

Recent critiques of hospital practices show that moral treatment needs to be revived. This is exemplified by a renewed concern with the practices of the therapeutic community, psychiatric clinics, and other similar community facilities.[33] What has been called a "social revolution" in the care of the mentally ill is, in many ways, a reintroduction of the fundamentals of the practice of humanitarian clinical care of the mentally ill as developed in the late 18th and early 19th centuries.

PSYCHOTHERAPEUTIC MOVEMENTS

Moral therapy played an integral role in the hospital treatment of the insane. An important aspect of this therapy was its emphasis on the relationship between the physician and the patient rather than the use of medical or surgical procedures. This principle has been recognized in the art of medicine since the time of the ancient Greeks, the patient's expectancies, faith, and attitude being crucial in the healing process, particularly concerning psychiatric disorders.

Early psychotherapies were often of a magico-religious nature, but in the 19th century psychotherapy began to be formalized and systematized. Following the methods of Mesmer,[34] hypnotic techniques were modified and applied to the treatment of psychoneurotic patients. Enthusiasm for the use of magnetism—or hypnosis, as Braid[35] termed it in 1843—occurred among many physicians and surgeons. It was repeatedly tried, at the time, for the treatment of the insane. The reports, however, were largely negative.[36] Hypnosis and suggestion became established as a psychotherapeutic procedure in the 1880s, largely through the efforts of Liebault, Charcot, and Bernheim. Bernheim elaborated on the concept of suggestibility, and reported his theories and treatment methods in his famous work *Suggestive Therapeutics*[37] that appeared in 1880. The dictum of the psychotherapy of 1880–1900 was that suggestion is everything, and Bernheim and his followers reported a number of successes, often declaring claims of 90% cure for various hysteric, psychosomatic, phobic, and depressive syndromes.

Table 2 summarizes reported results from various schools of psychotherapy. In his own work Bernheim reported 84% cures. Hypnosis was received with much enthusiasm, and some investigators, such as Voison,[38] reported favorable results in the treatment

TABLE 2

Results of Psychotherapy

Type of Therapy	No. of Cases	% Recovered & Markedly Improved
Bernheim (1887)	Hypnosis and Suggestion	50	84
Jacobson (1929)	Rest and Relaxation	79	77
Maudsley Hospital (1935)	Eclectic Psychotherapy	1,711	64
Ross (1936)	Eclectic Psychotherapy	1,089	77
Landis (1938)	Psychotherapy in Hospital	119	87
Knight (1941)	Psychoanalysis	660	56
Denker (1946)	General Practice	500	90
Miles (1951)	Psychoanalytic Psychotherapy	62	58
Brill & Beebe (1955)	Separation from Service	140	64
	Eclectic Psychotherapy	86	56
Wolpe (1958)	Behavior Therapy	210	90
Fact Finding Committee (Brody, 1962)	Psychoanalysis	210	60
Lazarus (1963)	Behavior Therapy	408	78
Marks and Gelder (1965)	Behavior Therapy	20	20
Heilbrunn (1966)	Psychoanalysis & Psychotherapy	173	45

of insanity, including melancholia. Its application was extended to many different conditions, such as organic brain disease, alcoholism, neuroses, and neuropathies, and was even applied to children for educational purposes. Richet, Janet, and others began to study hypnosis scientifically, with the result that a more moderate view was then expressed. Bernheim also became skeptical. By 1900 hypnosis was regarded as having questionable psychotherapeutic value. Referring to Bernheim, Janet stated: "The man who was always repeating that hypnotism was everything, now declares that hypnotism is nothing."[38]

The history of hypnosis has been one of waxing and waning, tremendous enthusiasm and overt rejection, as Janet has pointed out. This is largely true in relation to many of the psychotherapeutic schools introduced since Bernheim's time. It is likewise true of the rest cures of Weir Mitchell, the persuasive therapy of Dubois, the self-cure of Coué, the depth psychotherapies of Freud, Adler, and Jung with their many modifications, family therapy, conditioned reflex therapy, behavior therapy, exploratory psychotherapy, supportive psychotherapy, nondirective therapy, existential therapy, group psychotherapy, psychodrama, and group psychotherapeutic movements, such as Alcoholics Anonymous and Recovery.

Many movements similar to hypnosis emerge as a therapeutic revolution with a special vocabulary and a rallying about a charismatic leader with special healing powers. Personal training by the leader himself for the specific therapeutic method gives a special prowess and ability to the subsequent practitioner. Often when such movements begin, results of 90% or higher are presented; then a subsequent tempering of results and later rejection of the school occurs, particularly after the demise of the leader. Whatever has been proved valid in the movement finally becomes incorporated into the general body of psychiatric knowledge. Freud, repelled by the hypnotic and suggestive therapeutic practices of his day, aimed at establishing a scientifically sound and rational psychotherapy based on an etiologic theory of the psychoneuroses. Techniques of unconscious exploration, dream analysis, abreaction, free associations, interpretation, and use of the transference ensued. In the beginning, Freud had considerable belief in the efficacy of psychoanalysis; later, he admitted many doubts. In his *Introductory Lectures,* he rejected suggestion as the basis for the therapeutic results and analysis, pointing out that psychoanalysis produces results that are second to none of the finest in the field of internal medicine, and that these results could not have been achieved by any other procedure.[39] However, Freud never gave any statistical information to support this contention; he in fact rejected such methods. He believed that failures in therapy were due to an unsuitable choice of patients, the heterogeneous nature of psychiatric illness, plus the dangerous nature of transference, and, furthermore, the prejudices against him and psychoanalysis.

In the *New Introductory Lectures,*[40] Freud states that he was never a therapeutic enthusiast. After outlining again what he calls the uninstructive nature of statistics for evaluating psychoanalysis, he says: "I should like to add that I do not think our cures can compete with those of Lourdes. There are so many more people who believe in the miracles of the Blessed Virgin than in the existence of the unconscious." If we are to take Freud seriously here, he seems to imply that faith or belief in the unconscious is the prerequisite for cure in psychoanalysis. Following this reasoning to its logical conclusion, psychoanalysis then can be regarded as another form of faith healing. However, in comparison with other more mundane psychotherapeutic procedures, Freud concludes that psychoanalysis is beyond doubt the most powerful therapeutic method. Again he fails to present evidence along with comparative therapeutic data. In *Analysis Terminable and Interminable*,[41] he admits that his metapsychology could not be used to answer the limitations of analysis created by the strength of the instincts, the weakness of the ego, and the death instinct. Although admitting the limitations of analysis—its length, doubtful results, and problems in modifying the instincts and their defenses—Freud in no sense raises questions concerning his basic theories or therapeutic techniques. All this has earned him the unique position in the history of medicine of introducing a treatment modality that, as it developed, became lengthier, more expensive, and applicable to fewer and fewer patients—with ever more dubious results.

Knight[42] in 1941 summarized the few statistical studies of psychoanalysis (see Table 2) that in the treatment of psychoneuroses and some character neuroses recorded results of 56%. Unfortunately the Central Fact Finding Committee Report of the American Psychoanalytic Association has never published its findings because of reported methodologic problems.[43] These problems were due to a lack of uniformity in collecting data, resistance to completing questionnaires, and the number of patients listed as cured or markedly improved by one analyst but who later received treatment from another analyst. However, these deficiencies should not preclude a final report of the findings. Brody[44] reports from the study that of 595 psychoneurotic patients, 306 completed analysis but only 210 could be followed. Of these 210 cases, 80 were reported as cured, 46 as markedly improved, 74 improved, and a slight improvement was recognized in the remaining ten. Of those who completed treatment, Brody concludes that 97% were cured or improved. However, since the slightly improved and improved cases may reflect changes to be expected in the course of the neurosis, most investigators would not include these cases in the overall statistics, as has been done in Table 2. Summarizing the achievements of psychoanalysis, Brody states: "The 20th century has witnessed many advances in the treatment of emotional disorders but it is the accomplishments of psychoanalysis that stand at the cornerstone. Psychoanalysis has emerged not only as the most effective method known for the study of the human psyche, but as the most effective method known for the treatment of emotional disorders." Shortly after this, he adds: "Our science has not yet arrived at the point where we can statistically demonstrate its effectiveness. We have no criteria to determine degree of improvement."

Masserman,[45] who also reviewed the findings of the Central Fact Finding Committee, emphasized the need to reexamine the data, theories, and practices of psychoanalysis in the light of more fundamental scientific orientations. Heilbrunn,[46] reporting on the results of psychoanalysis and psychoanalytic-oriented therapy in private practice consisting of psychoneuroses, personality disorders, and a few mild psychotic patients, reported results of only 45% marked improvement. Without question, there is a greater need for such studies by individual practitioners, as to their own therapeutic efficiency, something that is surprisingly lacking in the psychiatric literature.

From Table 2, it can be noted that many differences in results have been reported in the use of various psychotherapeutic techniques. Jacobson,[47] whose techniques have never generally been followed by any group of psychiatrists, reported 77% improvement with relaxation methods. Denker[48] reported 90% improvement in treatment by the general practitioner. The Maudsley Hospital[49] and the careful study by Miles[50] show results respectively of 64% and 58%, which fall into the general percentage range of 60%–65%. Most investigators now believe this to be achievable in the treatment of psychoneuroses. Fiedler[51] made an interesting study in which he evaluated three different theoretic models, those of Freud, Adler, and Rogers. He concluded that the therapeutic results achieved did not differ, and that "the desirable therapeutic relationship is a function of the expertness of the therapist, rather than his theoretic orientation of therapeutic technique." Other surveys consistently have failed to reveal any overall differences in improvement rates with different theoretically oriented therapies.[52] Alexander[53] admits that the patient's faith in the therapy and the psychotherapist may be the most influential factor, rather than the therapist's theories, but he too fails to offer careful statistical studies. Glover[54] is a psychoanalyst who thinks that the main obstacle to subsequent developments in psychoanalysis has been the absence of reliable statistics and follow-up studies. The spontaneous remission rate in psychoneuroses is in need of more careful evaluation. Studies indicate that this rate may be between 40% and 60% improvement, thus indicating that nontherapeutic variables play a role in the course and outcome of psychoneuroses.[55]

In a recent and controversial review of the efficacy of psychotherapy, Eysenck concluded that untreated neurotic control groups, children as well as adults, recovered essentially to the same extent as those treated with psychotherapy.[56] His review stated that there is no indication that psychoanalytic psychotherapy, including formal psychoanalysis, has shown any greater effectiveness than eclectic psychotherapy. He does believe that techniques based on learning theory, such as those of Wolpe, lead to quicker and more general improvements than cases treated by eclectic or psychoanalytic psychotherapy. This recent technique has been reported as producing 90% results by Wolpe[57] and 78% results by Lazarus.[58] In fact, one Wolpe report claims that in studies of neurotic patients treated by nonpsychoanalytic methods, including his own, only four relapses occurred within a group of 249 patients—an incredible 98.8% improvement.[59] Such results are the closest to the reported figure of 100% recoveries claimed by Dr. William M. Awl ("Dr. Cure-Awl") in 1843.[9]

Is the behavior therapy a specific treatment method, or just another empirically oriented psychotherapy? Marks and Gelder,[60] in a carefully controlled study of behavior therapy, report improvement in only 60% of treated subjects and 50% of controls. The results for this treatment thus fall into the usual 60% range. There would seem to be merit, therefore, in any tendency to admit with Ackerknecht[61] that the therapeutic achievements based on psychodynamic and learning theories may not depend on any valid etiologic knowledge or on any causally oriented specific treatment. As some authors have stated,[62] therapy itself may be more closely related to mechanisms of suggestion, faith healing, social attitudes, and brainwashing. The favorable results may be largely dependent on patient nonspecific expectancy of relief, patient personality, social learning, and the skill, experience, and emotional attributes of the therapist rather than any current theoretic framework.[63]

THE REEMERGENCE OF PHYSICAL THERAPIES AND DRUGS

The concept of an organic deficit state in mental disorder, most likely involving the brain, is one that traces back to the days of Hippocrates. On the basis of this hypothesis a great number of

somatic therapies have been introduced. Man has made an eternal
search for means of tranquilization through both physical and
chemical means. Hydrotherapy, a means of physical tranquilization
used by the ancients, remained one of the principal means of con-
trolling patient overactivity until the advent of the newer somatic
therapies of the last 30 years. The continuous tub, cold packs,
douches, jet sprays, needle showers, colonic irrigation, the 50-degree
plunge, and other methods were used with varying degrees of
enthusiasm. In 1932 Wright[64] stated that, in the field of psychiatry,
hydrotherapy was a most important treatment method and should
be applied toward managing delirium, psychomotor excitement,
agitation, cerebral congestion, insomnia, and many other conditions.
Sedative, anodyne, hypnotic, eliminative, or stimulating effects can
be obtained through the hydriatric approach, but the days of
elaborate hydrotherapy procedures are nearly forgotten in this age
of chemotherapy.

Man has most intensively sought tranquilization through chemical means in such compounds as alcohol, hashish, and the opiates.
In the mid-18th century, Young[65] reported the dramatic therapeutic effects of opium for mania and melancholia. Brandeth regarded it as a specific for insanity, reporting that "large doses of
opium, in certain cases of insanity, have been frequently administered in many cases, with wonderful good effects."[66] During the
early 19th century, opiates were largely rejected. But by 1858
Bucknill and Tuke wrote: "The early writers on insanity condemned
the use of opiates and narcotics generally. They had not learned to
discriminate the conditions of mental disease in which opium becomes a true balm to the wounded spirit, a sedative in mania, a
restorative in melancholia; sometimes even a tonic. . . . The opiate
treatment has gradually undergone development, until, at the present time, the skillful and discriminating use of this drug may be
truly called the sheet anchor of the alienist physician."[67] In the mid-
19th century opium was at the zenith of its use, but the recognition
of its addicting qualities led to its rejection by the end of the
century.[68]

The search for the ideal tranquilizer has been a lengthy one.
Many drugs have appeared and disappeared over the last 100 years,
but the greatest plethora of drugs has occurred within the past 15
years. Drugs have been used as hypnotics, to calm excited patients,
and to relieve disturbing symptoms such as anxiety and depression.
Stimulants also have been used in attempts to activate apathetic,

retarded, and depressed patients. Drugs have functioned as forms of restraint and have been combined with humane treatment and psychotherapy. The more popular drugs of the early 19th century included tartrate of antimony, hellebore, ipecac, digitalis, calomel, and quinine. In the 1850s the bromides were introduced[69] and used for sedative purposes, having great popularity until the 1890s. Hyoscyamus, belladonna, cannabis indica, and conium all had their heyday, only to be forgotten. Chloral was developed and used in 1869,[70] paraldehyde in 1882,[71] cannabis indica in 1880, and the barbiturates in 1903.[72] Again these were introduced with waves of enthusiasm, but their limited value was observed over the years. Nevertheless, a number of these continue to be important compounds for the psychiatrist.

Many physical treatment measures that made their appearance have disappeared, such as oophorectomy, castration, hysterectomy, trephining, removal of various organs for focal infection, fever therapy, and, later, lobotomy. Nutritional, metabolic, and endocrinologic approaches have been developed. From these approaches came three remarkable conquests. In 1891 Murray[73] reported on the successful treatment of myxedema by hypodermic injections of sheep thyroid-gland extract. Goldberger in 1914[74] reported on the treatment and prevention of pellagra by diet, and finally in 1938 niacin[75] was isolated and identified. In 1887 Wagner von Jauregg[76] experimented with fever therapy, noticing that it had no consistent effect on the insane. He did, nonetheless, introduce fever therapy by the inoculation of malaria for general paresis in 1917,[77] a treatment method that could arrest the disease process. With Fleming's introduction of penicillin[78] and Mahoney's[79] demonstration of its specific antiluetic action, general paresis was essentially conquered. In the area of myxedema and cretinism, pellagra, and general paresis, achievements in psychiatry have remained a paradigm for investigation of other psychiatric disorders, since these have been made with a basic understanding of cause, and with specific treatment and means of prevention.

Hopes of similar achievement in the treatment of schizophrenia were expressed by Sakel, Meduna, and Moniz in the development in the 1930s of their somatic therapies: insulin, electroconvulsive therapy, and lobotomy. These individuals were clinicians who worked in psychiatric hospitals rather than research laboratories, and sought empiric treatments for their patients. Though their hopes never were fully realized, their therapeutic methods demonstrated some degree of efficacy. Perhaps most important of all, they changed the generally prevailing attitude of pessimism, particularly toward schizophrenia. Today, however, insulin therapy is rarely used in the treatment of schizophrenia, but is accepted as having its greatest value in the treatment of manic-depressive and involutional-depressive illnesses.

Insulin therapy, the first of the modern somatotherapies, was utilized by Sakel from 1927 to 1933, and was introduced in the literature as a treatment for schizophrenia in 1934.[80] Insulin increased the appetite and weight of patients, as well as producing a sedative effect. After its initial application in the treatment of the excitement and agitation of morphine withdrawal in cases of addiction, it seemed only logical that it be applied to schizophrenia, where appetite disturbances and agitation are such common symptoms. The theory of the treatment was based on the hypothesis that through the intensification of parasympathetic activity, blockading the nerve cells, and strengthening anabolism, the endogenously deranged nerve cells of the schizophrenics would be restored and the patient presumably would recover from his illness. Sakel believed he had discovered a specific treatment for schizophrenia by administering insulin to produce a state of hypoglycemic coma, which he called the Sakel Classical Insulin Shock Treatment. He felt his treatment was curative, and in his initial reports (see Table 3) he spoke of 88% improvement in acute cases.[81]

Sakel[82] continued to champion his treatment throughout his life despite the many resistances to his therapy and the failure of psychiatrists to pursue his highly specific technique. Against a staggering number of reports that failed to support his thesis, he again and again emphasized that results of 90% cure or marked improvement could be obtained. By 1939 the New York State Hospital Study[83] of the Sakel concept reported immediate results of 59%; Rennie[84] and later Bond,[85] results of 55%; and Gottlieb and Huston,[86] results of 35%. Follow-up studies showed that with the passing of time there was an increased rate of relapse. In response to these more limited results, Sakel stated: "Successful results, achieved by my students in various hospitals, ranged from 2 per cent to 37.1 per cent. Not one—not even the most successful of the contributors—attacked the percentages of successful and fully authenticated cures that I had achieved"; and furthermore: "Even if the Sakel Insulin Method should not remain the final answer to the problem of mental disease, it has proved itself up to now the most

TABLE 3

Insulin Therapy of Schizophrenia

	% Recovered or Markedly Improved
Dussik and Sakel (1936)	
Recent Cases	88
Subacute Cases	48
Muller (1937)	70
Malzberg (1938)	65
Ross and Malzberg (1939)	
Recent Cases	59
Subacute Cases	51
Chronic Cases	38
Rennie (1943)	
Immediate Response	55
at 3-yr Follow-up	33
Bond (1944)	
Immediate Response	55
at 4-yr Follow-up	33
Gottlieb and Huston (1951)	35
Staudt and Hoch (1957)	
Immediate Response	58
at 1-yr Follow-up	46
at 2 to 5-yr Follow-up	30–40
Spontaneous Remission Rate, Pre-shock	
(Staudt and Hoch, 1957)	30–40

valuable tool for a successful physiopsychologic approach to the problem of mental disease."[82]

However, with such inconclusive and contradictory evidence relative to the efficacy of insulin therapy, and with the introduction of the psychopharmacologic agents in psychiatry, the demise of insulin-coma therapy was inevitable. As Ackner et al,[87] in their provocative study, remarked: "No conclusion can be drawn about the therapeutic value of the coma regime, but the results suggest that insulin is not the specific therapeutic agent." Bond[88] in his follow-up studies reported initial favorable results of 63%, but a relapse rate of 44% of these improved cases in one month, and a 78% relapse rate in one year. Bond admits that although insulin therapy was effective in restoring the schizophrenic patient to his prepsy-chotic adjustment, it was not accompanied by a permanent correction of factors that led to the development of the illness.[89] In 1960 Hoff, who was closely identified at the outset with insulin treatment, stated: "It is quite possible that the time is approaching, and it may be quite soon, when the insulin treatment will no longer be used."[90] Sakel's achievement seems to rest not with his introduction and struggle for the acceptance of insulin therapy but in the impetus he gave to the biologic aspects of psychiatric research.

Meduna introduced convulsive therapy in 1934,[91] basing its development on the fallacious hypothesis that there is a negative relationship between epilepsy and schizophrenia. Clinicians had made occasional observations for some time that isolated patients with insanity apparently had improved when they suffered a convulsion. Initially camphor and later Metrazol were used to induce the convulsions.

Meduna was convinced that he had originated a valuable new treatment for schizophrenia; his initial reports were 52% and later 60% recovery or marked improvement. In 1938 Sorger and Hoffman,[92] on the basis of their treatment of 100 cases, reported that Metrazol treatment had produced remissions in schizophrenia amounting to 100% in acute amentiform conditions, 81% in acute and subacute stupor, 71% in acute and subacute hebephrenia, and 68% in acute and subacute paranoid-hallucinatory conditions. Such encouraging reports were not to be followed, although as late as 1944 Cook[93] claimed 70% recovery or marked improvement.

The replacement of chemical inducement of convulsions by the use of electric current was a logical one. After a lengthy series of animal experiments, Cerletti and Bini[94] in 1938 produced the first induced electric convulsion in man. Meduna, Cerletti, and Bini emphasized that the critical factor in treatment was the convulsion and not the chemical or the electric factor. Because of added convenience, better control, and reduced patient anxiety, electroconvulsive therapy (ECT) became the common method of treatment. The ease of application soon led to its widespread use. Kalinowsky's[95] early reports of 67% recovery or marked improvement and those of Cook[93] of 70% positive results stimulated extensive use of ECT in the treatment of schizophrenia. Over a period of time investigators lost interest; often the reported period of improvement was very transitory, and any value greater than the spontaneous remission rate was questionable (see Table 4). At the present time this therapy is being used in relatively few cases of schizophrenia. Five-year follow-up studies with both insulin and convulsive thera-

TABLE 4

Convulsive Therapies for Schizophrenia

		% Recovered or Markedly Improved
Metrazol		
Meduna (1938)		52
Kuppers (1938)		53
Meduna and Friedman (1939)		
	Acute Cases	60
	Subacute Cases	52
Pollack (1939)		34
Reznikoff (1940)		
	Immediate Response	44
	at 1-yr Follow-up	32
Cook (1944)		
	Acute Cases	70
ECT		
Kalinowsky and Worthing (1943)		
	Acute Cases	67
	Subacute Cases	43
Cook (1944)		
	Acute Cases	68
Lowinger and Huddleson (1946)		
	Acute Cases	54
	Subacute Cases	40
Gottlieb and Huston (1951)		46
Staudt and Zubin (1957)		52
Spontaneous Remission Rate, Pre-shock		
	(Staudt and Zubin, 1957)	30–40

pies show that the differences in therapeutic results between treated groups and controls are only slightly in favor of those treated.[96]

In 1937 Verstraeten[97] reported on the use of Metrazol convulsive therapy in the treatment of manic-depressive disease. Since then it has been proved that in manic-depressive and involutional-depressive diseases, convulsive therapy produces definite and consistent therapeutic results. This is illustrated in the carefully controlled studies of Huston,[98] where improvement of 81% is reported for involutional illnesses and 82% in manic-depressive illness.[99] Bond[88] obtained similar results but emphasized that the value of convulsive therapy in manic-depressive illness was largely one of reducing the duration of the attack rather than preventing subsequent attacks. ECT remains the most effective treatment for severe depressive psychoses.

In 1933 Egas Moniz conceived the idea of prefrontal lobotomy for schizophrenic patients. This idea had its foundation in the theory of disturbed synaptic paths between the prefrontal lobes and the thalamus. On the basis of cytoarchitectonic charts, Moniz postulated that because the higher psychic functions are localized in the prefrontal cortex, this area must be primarily disturbed in schizophrenia. He thus decided to sever the connecting paths to the prefrontal cortex, which in turn would transform the patient's psychic reactions. The first operation was performed in 1935. Egas Moniz[100] stated that both cures and improvements resulted. Freeman and Watts[101] popularized this procedure in the United States despite many critical opinions, emphasizing the very favorable results obtained. In a follow-up study of a 10-to-20-year period of 500 prefrontal lobotomies, Freeman and Watts[102] reported a discharge rate of from 70% to 80% for schizophrenia, with 40% to 50% of patients being favorably employed. With the transorbital lobotomy, the results were even more amazing: a five-year follow-up study showed 87% discharges and 70% employed. Although other investigators have reported favorable results, with time and the introduction of new methods of treatment lobotomy is very rarely used today for the treatment of schizophrenia. It is worthy of note that no other investigators[103] were able to achieve the results presented by Freeman and Watts.

As has been indicated in this review, most therapeutic developments and movements have been simplistically identified and made synonymous with a particular person—eg, hypnosis with Mesmer; moral therapy with Pinel and Tuke; nonrestraint with Conolly; hospital planning with Kirkbride; suggestion with Liebault and Bernheim; psychoanalysis with Freud; fever therapy with Wagner von Jauregg; insulin coma therapy with Sakel; convulsive therapy with Meduna, Cerletti, and Bini; lobotomy with Egas Moniz; and behavior therapy with Wolpe. On the other hand, the two most recent developments in psychiatry—psychopharmacotherapy and community psychiatry—are not strongly identified with any particular individual or school. The former is the result of combined research by the pharmaceutic industry, universities, National Institute of Mental Health, and the Food and Drug Administration; the latter is a social and political action.

The modern era of psychopharmacology began in 1951 with the French scientist Laborit's[104] synthesis of chlorpromazine (Thorazine), which was originally intended for use in the management of general anesthesia. It was described as a vagolytic, sympathicolytic, spasmolytic, antipyretic, antiemetic, and sedative. Soon thereafter, Delay's and Deniker's[105] still valid clinical appraisal was applied throughout Europe to all types of disorders in which vegetative disturbances occur, such as anxiety states, agitated depressions, deliria, mania, and schizophrenia. By 1954 chlorpromazine and reserpine were in the forefront of psychiatric discussions on the North American continent. Since then the literature on these and related phenothiazines has mounted to thousands of articles. In 1954 it was predicted that these compounds would soon replace insulin and the convulsive therapies in schizophrenia, a prediction that essentially was realized within a few years' time. Many spectacular reports were made of the efficacy of these drugs in the relief of psychotic excitement, agitation, hallucinations, anxiety, and related symptoms. Early, Kinross-Wright[106] reported remission or marked improvement in 68 of 95 patients. On chronic psychotic patients, Borsa and Kline[107] reported improvements in 84% of 740 patients with reserpine; 150 patients reached such a level of improvement that they were able to leave the hospital. Within two years chlorpromazine was well established as a valuable therapeutic agent.

Chlorpromazine was regarded as being palliative rather than curative by most investigators.[108] After the experiences of curative results and spectacular improvements with insulin, convulsive therapy, and lobotomy, investigators tended to be more conservative in their approach. They were enthusiastic and hopeful, but emphasized the need for careful methodologies, strict self-criticism, and the use of control and double-blind studies. Results have been impressively presented for the usefulness of chlorpromazine. Winkleman[109] described 84% effectiveness as compared with 34% with a placebo, and Denker and Bird[110] reported 81.8% improvement in 1,523 cases. After a five-year follow-up, Winkleman[111] reported a continued remission or marked improvement in 75% of his cases. With the use of a number of different psychotropic drugs there has been a decline reported in state hospital populations, indicating the value of the new treatments,[112] particularly among schizophrenic patients. Though problems with younger and older groups of patients, as well as future relapses in schizophrenic patients, may offset these gains, no similar decline in patient populations co-incided with the introduction of insulin and convulsive therapies. A few studies do not support the trend of hospital-population patient reduction.[113] In addition, chlorpromazine and other ataractic drugs have been used in combination with psychotherapy, milieu therapy, and other techniques, their soundness and application having been well documented. Maintenance therapy has been used for lengthy periods, with relapses being common when the drug is discontinued.

Iproniazid (Marsilid), which was observed to induce euphoria in tubercular patients, was applied to depressive illnesses in 1954[114] with some success—and thus began the second great psychophar-macologic movement involving the antidepressant drugs. Its action as a monoamine oxidase inhibitor (MAO) has been studied, and many similarly acting compounds without the toxicity of iproniazid have been introduced in the treatment of depression. Several years later imipramine (Tofrānil),[115] and later amitriptyline (Elavil)[116] and other tricyclic drugs, believed to sensitize central adrenergic mechanisms at the synaptic level, were introduced as a treatment for depression. Their efficacy in controlled studies has been by now clearly demonstrated. They have led to a great reduction of the use of convulsive therapies in the treatment of the depressive illnesses. However, ECT leads to a higher degree of rapid improvement in many instances, especially in psychiatric emergencies, and by no means has been replaced by antidepressive medication.[117]

Since the mid-fifties, so many new antipsychotic, antidepressive, and anti-anxiety drugs have been developed that it has been impos-sible for most psychiatrists to keep abreast of the information ex-plosion. These compounds, synthesized primarily by chemists asso-ciated with the pharmaceutic industry, are evaluated on animals, after which the psychiatrist performs clinical human evaluation. Through the manipulation of certain basic molecular structures known to have psychoactive properties, a seemingly infinite number of compounds can be produced. The goal has been to seek those with maximum therapeutic efficacy and minimum side reactions. The pharmaceutic industry sponsors scientific meetings to report on and promote their products, with other less dramatic incentives and severest critical appraisals emanating from research divisions in mental hospitals, university psychiatric departments, and govern-ment agencies. With one fourth to one third of all prescriptions now being written for psychoactive drugs, we are in the great age of psychopharmacology, in which industry has great stakes. Compounds that may have considerable therapeutic value but no presumed potential for commercial exploration, such as the use of lithium salts in mania,[118] were at first not presented seriously to the psychiatric profession. The physician has become increasingly dependent on brochures from drug companies rather than formal scientific reports. As Wortis[119] emphasized: "Intense competition among companies leads not only to valuable discoveries of new products, but also to a confusing and superfluous variety, which in turn entails an enormous promotional activity that is bound to exaggerate the positive and minimize the negative features of a product."

Fortunately, during the past 12 years the situation has improved. The most exacting scrutiny aimed at the evaluation of the many psychoactive drugs is now made by the Psychopharmacology Research Branch of the National Institute of Mental Health and the Food and Drug Administration. Psychopharmacology has brought psychiatry and medicine closer together, with an emphasis on investigation into biochemical and enzymatic dysfunction in psychiatric disorders. Collaborative studies of a number of hospitalized patients, sponsored by the Psychopharmacology Research Branch of the National Institute of Mental Health, have revealed the value of medications through carefully controlled studies. No one drug studied was found to be significantly superior to another in the treatment of schizophrenia. The nonspecific antipsychotic effect of the phenothiazines[120] is a case in point. The carefully controlled quality and methodology of these studies offers a welcome addition to psychiatric studies in general. The anti-anxiety drugs, similarly under controlled conditions, show no specificity, but these do relieve anxiety. There is present a question of drug dependency relative to minor tranquilizers, a problem the Food and Drug Administration has under study. Pragmatically, the value of the drugs over the past ten years has undoubtedly been reflected in a statistically significant decrease in the number of patients in psychiatric hospitals, resulting in an increase of their care within the community. The tremendous implications for psychiatry in the light of these developments in psychopharmacology and neurobiology recently were summarized by Elkes as follows:

> . . . For I know of no other branch of science which, like a good plough on a spring day, has tilled as many areas as neurobiology. To have, in a mere decade, questioned the concepts of synaptic transmission in the central nervous system; to have emphasized compartmentalization and regionalization of chemical process in

the unit cell, and in the brain; to have focused on the interaction of hormone and chemical process within the brain; to have given us tools for the study of the chemical basis of learning and temporary connection formation; to have emphasized the dependence of pharmacological response on its situational and social setting; to have compelled a hard look at the semantics of psychiatric diagnosis, description and communication; to have resuscitated that oldest of old remedies, the placebo response, for careful scrutiny; to have provided potential methods for the study of language in relation to the functional state of the brain; and to have encouraged the biochemist, physiologist, psychologist, clinician, and the mathematician and communication engineer to join forces at bench level, is no mean achievement for a young science. That a chemical text should carry the imprint of experience, and partake in its growth, in no way invalidates study of the symbols and the rules among symbols, which keep us going, changing, evolving and human.

Thus, though moving cautiously from set habit to positive scepticism, psychopharmacology is still protesting; yet, in so doing it is, for the first time, compelling the physical and chemical sciences to look behavior in the face, and thus enriching both the science and behavior. If there be discomfiture in this encounter, it is hardly surprising; for it is in this discomfiture that there may well lie the germ of a new science.[121]

COMMUNITY PSYCHIATRY

Hailed as the third psychiatric revolution[122] or dismissed as the latest therapeutic bandwagon,[123] the current trend in psychiatric treatment is a mammoth encompassing program and corporate effort known as community psychiatry. Emphasis on understanding has shifted from the individual patient to the family, social, and cultural milieu. Such interests revert to the early decades of the 19th century when the influence of society, its culture, organization, institutions, industrialization, and calamities were related to mental illness. Mental illness then was considered to be increasing due to the rise of civilization, and man's "excess passion for liberty."[14] Burrows[124] believed in the social causation of mental illness and was optimistic about its treatment. Brigham,[125] analyzing the increase of insanity in 1832, reported four contributing factors: first, too constant and too powerful excitement of the mind, which the strife for wealth, office, political distinction, and party success produces in this free country; second, the predominance given to the nervous system by too early cultivating the mind and exciting the feelings of children; third, neglect of physical education, or the equal and proper development of all organs of the body; fourth, the general and powerful excitement of the female mind. In 1857 Hawkes[24] wrote of the need to apply the general principles of prevention to mental illnesses through social action and reform.

However, not until the early 20th century were the roots of community psychiatry evident in the work of Clifford Beers and Adolph Meyer. In 1909 the mental hygiene movement was initiated; sociologic and epidemiologic studies relating mental disorder to social instability began in the 1920s; the Commonwealth Fund support for the first Child Guidance Clinics came in 1922. A Mental Health Division in the United States Public Health Service was established in 1930; the accumulation of psychiatric experiences in World War II resulted in the development of the National Institute of Mental Health in 1947.

Community psychiatry is to be viewed as a social action movement, largely influenced by public pressures, political forces, and legislative measures at the local, state, and particularly the federal level. Its theoretic bases are the knowledge gained from the social and behavioral sciences rather than from the specialty of psychiatry within the discipline of medicine. The traditional doctor-patient (one-to-one) relationship is transcended, with the shift in diagnosis and therapy to the family and the community. Modern conventional psychiatry, exemplified in private practice, has of late isolated itself from the general domain of medicine and the community just as hospital psychiatry isolated itself 80 years ago.[126] The psychodynamic model and its individual approach in many ways has been limited in offering solutions and proving its usefulness for the masses. The effort to attain full potential is sought through community mental health centers, which aim at primary prevention and at treatment of existing cases, often referred to as secondary prevention. Many of the present-day principles are not new. They have been exemplified in many mental hospitals although never applied so widely as now.

Further impetus toward the development of community psychiatry has come from the ever-widening definition of mental illness, which tends to include delinquents, sex offenders, addicts, alcoholics, and many different types of political extremists. Also included are those areas of neglect embracing the mentally retarded, the chronic psychotics, and the senile degeneratives.

Community psychiatry incorporates many therapeutic techniques into its armamentarium, a large number of which rest on the previously practiced humanitarian traditions of the past. As stated in *Action for Mental Health:*

> To Pinel's principles for the treatment of psychotics twentieth-century psychiatry can add little, except to convert them into modern terminological dress, contribute more systematic thought on the significance of various symptoms, intensify the doctor-patient relationship through scientific knowledge of psychological mechanisms, treat the patient as a member of a social group which expects him to behave in accepted ways, and specify that moral treatment has been subject to an incredible amount of distortion and misinterpretation depending on the personality, motivations and vicissitudes of its administrators.[127]

Community psychiatry, incorporating many psychiatric approaches toward the alleviation of emotional suffering, must be selective in its orientation to patient care. Accepting that a psychiatric disorder is intimately related to the social milieu, we observe within the framework of the hospital and clinic the development of the therapeutic community—or milieu therapy—which has been defined as "a scientific manipulation of the environment aimed at producing changes in the personality of the patient."[128] The intent is to help the patient regain a positive relation to his family and community environment. To do so incorporates appropriate use of drugs, and group and individual psychotherapy, with sustained contact wherever possible rather than isolation from family and community.

Emphasis is placed therefore on treatment in the community, the utilization of clinic resources, day and night hospital units, crisis-oriented therapy, rehabilitation and aftercare, hospitalization in psychiatric units in general hospitals, earlier discharge, use of half-way houses, and the establishment of special programs for the mentally retarded, aged, alcoholics, and addicts. The education of the public regarding mental illness becomes paramount in helping change community attitudes toward the mentally ill. Work with schools, clinics, various agencies, and churches is therefore another important aspect of the program. The psychiatrist's role thus has shifted from the doctor-patient relationship to that of community leader and educator; direct work with patients is often relegated to the social worker, nurse, psychologist, and others.

What are the therapeutic results of these community mental health programs in terms of treatment of cases and prevention of mental illness? Although programs have been extensively developed, results remain largely impressionistic, as patient discharges are divided into the community (transfers to family care), chronic hospitals, and other institutions. The recent *Milbank Memorial Fund Quarterly* report[129] attempts an initial presentation of evaluation studies regarding the effectiveness of community mental health services. Most data presented in these reports focus on a description of programs, general statistical data—including numbers of patients seen—diagnoses, referral sources, discharges, etc., with minimal emphasis on therapeutic results in terms of clinical change. Binner,[130] reviewing the figures for discharged patients at the Fort Logan Program during the first three years of operation, reported 39% of cases as recovered or markedly improved, 28% as slightly improved. Interestingly, for the 1961/62 cohort, the recovery and markedly improved rate was 53%; for 1962/63, 38%; and for 1963/64 it had fallen to 32%. This phenomenon is similar to that described by Earle in the early hospital movement—namely, an initial high rate of recovery and marked improvement, with a subsequent gradual decline. Binner relates this decline to a number of factors, such as early therapeutic enthusiasm, different clinicians' ratings, change in composition of patient population, and variations in period of hospitalization. Data from other centers with follow-up studies is urgently needed before extensive programs are launched that may not necessarily fulfill the expected hopes of the community psychiatry enthusiasts.

Confusion still exists as to the differentiating point between mental illness and mental health. There is need for strict evaluation of the problems of illness with favorable therapeutic change versus discharge into the community without any basic change. For instance, how often do discharges occur due to administrative needs rather than favorable results? Are these programs helping patients to function better when assimilated into the community, or is there some alteration of basic psychopathologic processes?

Ascertaining the value of preventive methods is extremely difficult, and no satisfactory criteria have been established. There are many sweeping and fundamental forces that create society's problems, complex historic and cultural factors that seem beyond control in terms of our current knowledge and the application of that knowledge. Wars, interracial strife, technologic progress, economic rises and declines, urbanization, disintegrating communities, and population growth—such forces, fundamentally social and political, remain beyond the province and means of the psychiatrist. Burrows expressed considerable wisdom when he stated in 1828 that "great political and civil revolutions in states are always productive of great enthusiasm in the people. In proportion as the feelings are acted upon, so will insanity be more or less frequent."[124] If we widen his definition of insanity to include the patient groups of today, we must agree with this basic premise.

As we know, literally millions of dollars are being expended on the community programs, with great claims for potential success being heralded throughout the nation. But the fundamental question remains: How can our present knowledge effectively develop such programs? As a result of some of our mythology about therapy, together with a political belief that we can legislate away the problems of man, are we about to enter a second "cult of curability" rather than a "third psychiatric revolution"? Should the psychiatrist enter into the power structure of the community, and if so, to what extent? Or should he function primarily in the more direct treatment of patients? Further accumulation of knowledge through controlled and scientifically designed research seems imperative before we can more fully understand the complexity of human behavior, and thus develop specific therapeutic approaches as well as extend the potential of the great moral tradition in psychiatry.

CONCLUSION

The need to maintain a historic perspective in approaching current psychiatric developments has been emphasized in this presentation. Since the introduction of the great humanitarian-treatment tradition in psychiatry over 150 years ago, there has been a waxing and waning of interests and reports of therapeutic efficacy. High rates of curability for insanity, often reaching 90%, were reported with the moral therapy and hospitalization during the first half of the 19th century. By the 1870s there was an attitude of therapeutic nihilism for the insane. Before the end of the century, psychiatry, through the efforts of the hypnotists and Freud, focused on the psychoneuroses, and great claims were made for the effectiveness of psychotherapy. Since 1900 many schools of psychiatry and psychotherapy have been developed through sundry charismatic leaders, their theories, and followers. Meanwhile, significant discoveries were being made and specific treatment measures developed for certain endocrine disorders (cretinism and myxedema), pellagra, and general paresis.

Psychiatry began to shift increasingly from the mental hospital to the clinic and private practice, with optimism in the treatment of the neuroses and a continuing pessimistic therapeutic attitude toward the psychoses. The 1930s saw the development of new treatments for the psychotics in the somatic therapies. As the therapeutic attitude toward patients changed, remarkable results were reported for the somatic therapies: insulin coma, convulsive therapy, and lobotomy. Two broad schools of psychiatry emerged, the organic-physical treatment oriented, and the psychodynamic-psychotherapeutic group. The former focused on psychotic patients, and the latter largely on the psychoneurotic and characteriologic problems. As the limitations of both the somatic and psychotherapeutic techniques have gradually been realized, measures of modification and new schools of treatment have continued to emerge. Presently the somatic therapies of the 1930s survive almost solely in the application of electroconvulsive therapy for the treatment of depressions. No etiology-oriented specific treatment measures were discovered.

Since the early 1950s there have been two significant developments: psychopharmacology and community psychiatry. The age of psychopharmacology has produced many remarkable symptomatic treatment measures, but again no specific treatments. Methods of determining values of psychiatric therapies have come to the fore because of the many drugs introduced, leading to previously nonexistent sophisticated techniques of evaluation. Impetus to study further the biologic bases of behavior has resulted from this work on drugs and behavior, a movement closely associated with the pharmaceutical industry and not identified with any particular individual or any special school of psychiatry.

The second development, which has led to a changing role for the psychiatrist, has been one of social action, demanded by public needs and executed through legislative means. The community psychiatry movement has been repeatedly accoladed as the third psychiatric revolution, and millions of dollars—local, state, and federal—are being expended for its development. In many ways this movement is a reemphasis of the humanitarian tradition introduced 150 years ago; many of its methods, regarded as unique, were defined although not realized over 100 years ago. Knowledge regarding the results of these programs continues to be very vague and incomplete; careful evaluations are imperative. The movement, based on humanitarian beliefs rather than being causally or scientifically oriented, leaves much in doubt as to the etiology and treatment of mental disorder. Furthermore, confusion and complexity are added because of the widening definition of mental illness.

In our desire to achieve therapeutic results we must not succumb to the premise that humanitarianism in itself is the solution to our psychiatric problems. Knowledge as to cause, course, psychopathology, or pathophysiology remains lacking for the majority of psychiatric disorders. Treatments, therefore, regardless of the therapeutic intent, remain symptomatic and nonspecific. Has another "cult of curability" been created, or are we truly in the throes of a great psychiatric revolution? Are we to founder in the mire of social application and propaganda before the establishment of a hard basis of fact?

REFERENCES

1. Pinel, P.: *Treatise on Insanity,* D. D. Davis (trans.), Sheffield: W. Todd, 1806.
2. Tuke, S.: *Description of the Retreat, An Institution Near York for Insane Persons,* York: W. Alexander, 1813.
3. Esquirol, J. E. D.: *Mental Maladies: Treatise on Insanity,* E. K. Hunt (trans.), Philadelphia: Lee and Blanchard, 1845.
4. Haslam, J.: *Observations on Insanity, with Practical Remarks on the Disease, and Account of Morbid Appearances on Dissection,* London: F. and C. Rivington, 1798.
5. *Report from Committee Appointed to Examine Physicians Who Have Attended His Majesty, During His Illness, Touching on the State of His Majesty's Health, 1788,* printed by the Order of the House of Commons, 10 December 1788.
6. Ray, I.: Statistics of Insane Hospitals, *Amer. J. Insanity,* 6:23, 1849–1850.
7. Burrows, G. M.: *Inquiry Into Certain Errors Relative to Insanity; and their Consequences, Physical, Moral and Civil,* London: Thomas and Underwood, 1820.
8. Hall, B.: *Travels in North America in the Years 1827 and 1828,* Philadelphia, 1829.
9. Deutsch, A.: *The Mentally Ill in America,* ed. 2, New York: Columbia University Press, 1949.
10. Kirkbride, T. S.: Remarks on Construction, Organization and General Arrangements of Hospitals for Insane, *Amer. J. Insanity,* 11:1, 18, 1854–1855.
11. Butler, J. S.: *Curability of Insanity and Individualized Treatment of the Insane,* New York: G. P. Putnam's Sons, 1887.
12. Grob, G. N.: Samuel B. Woodward and the Practice of Psychiatry in Early Nineteenth-Century America, *Bull. Hist. Med.,* 36:420, 1962.
13. Conolly, J.: *Treatment of Insane Without Mechanical Restraints,* London: Smith, Elder and Co., 1856.

14. Rush, B.: *Medical Inquiries and Observations Upon Diseases of the Mind,* Philadelphia: Kimber and Richardson, 1812.
15. Statistical Reports. Lunatic Asylums in the United States, *Amer. J. Insanity,* 2:46, 1845.
16. Summary of Statistics of American Hospitals for Insane, *Amer. J. Insanity,* 17:317, 1861.
17. Earle, P.: *Curability of Insanity,* Philadelphia: J. B. Lippincott, 1887.
18. Earle, P.: *History, Description and Statistics of Bloomingdale Asylum of Insane,* New York: Egberg, Honey and King, 1849.
19. Bockoven, J. S.: *Moral Treatment in American Psychiatry,* New York, Springer Publishing Co., 1963.
20. (a) Gray, J. P.: Dependence of Insanity on Physical Disease, *Amer. J. Insanity,* 27:377, 1871.
    (b) Gray, J. P.: Insanity: Its Frequency and Some of Its Preventable Causes, *Amer. J. Insanity,* 42:1, 1885–1886.
21. Kirkbride, T. S.: *On Organization and General Arrangement of Hospitals for the Insane with Some Remarks on Insanity and Its Treatment,* ed. 2, Philadelphia: J. B. Lippincott, 1880.
22. Earle, P.: Prospective Provision for Insane, *Amer. J. Insanity,* 25:51, 1868.
23. Bartemeir, L. H., Appel, K. E., Ewalt, J. E., and Barton, W. E.: Future of Psychiatry: Report of Joint Commission on Illness and Health, *Amer. J. Psychiat.,* 118:973, 1962.
24. Hawkes, J.: On Increase of Insanity, *J. Psychol. Med. and Ment. Path.,* 10:508, 1857.
25. Dain, N.: *Concepts of Insanity in the United States, 1789–1865,* New Brunswick: Rutgers University Press, 1964.
26. Allen, M.: *Essay on Classification of Insane,* London: Taylor, 1837.
27. Ellis, W. C.: *Treatise on Nature, Symptoms, Causes, and Treatment of Insanity, with Practical Observations on Lunatic Asylums,* London: Holdsworth, 1838.
28. Seymour, J. S.: *Thoughts on Nature and Treatment of Several Severe Diseases of Human Body,* London: Longmans, 1847.
29. Arlidge, J. T.: *On States of Lunacy and Legal Provision for the Insane, with Observations on Construction and Organization of Asylums,* London: Churchill, 1859.
30. Gaskell, S.: On Want of Better Provision for Labouring and Middle Classes When Attacked or Threatened with Insanity, *J. Ment. Sci.,* 6:321, 1860.
31. Ozarin, L. D.: Moral Treatment and the Mental Hospital, *Amer. J. Psychiat.,* 111:371, 1954.
32. Hurd, H. M. (ed.): *Institutional Care of Insane in the United States and Canada,* vol. 1, Baltimore: Johns Hopkins Press, 1916.
33. (a) Jones, M.: *Therapeutic Community,* New York: Basic Books, 1953.
    (b) Stanton, A., and Schwartz, M.: *The Mental Hospital,* New York: Basic Books, 1954.
    (c) Greenblatt, M., York, R. H., and Brown, E. L.: *From Custodial to Therapeutic Care in Mental Hospitals,* New York: Russell Sage Foundation, 1955.
    (d) Dunham, H. W. and Weinberg, N. S.: *Culture of the State Mental Hospital,* Detroit: Wayne State University Press, 1960.
34. Mesmer, F. A.: *Mesmerism* (trans. from *Mémoire sur la découverte du Magnétisme Animal*), London: Macdonald, 1948.
35. Braid, J.: *Neurypnology, or Rationale of Nervous Sleep,* London: J. Churchill, 1843.

36. Galt, J. M.: *Treatment of Insanity,* New York: Harper and Brothers, 1846.
37. Bernheim, H.: *Suggestive Therapeutics: Treatise on Nature and Uses of Hypnotism,* New York: G. P. Putnam's Sons, 1880.
38. Janet, P.: *Psychological Healing: Historical and Clinical Study,* New York: Macmillan, 1925.
39. Freud, S.: "Introductory Lectures on Psychoanalysis," in *Standard Edition of Complete Psychological Works,* vols. 15, 16, London: Hogarth Press, 1963.
40. Freud, S.: "New Introductory Lectures on Psychoanalysis," in *Standard Edition of Complete Psychological Works,* vol. 22, London: Hogarth Press, 1964, pp. 1–182.
41. Freud, S.: "Analysis Terminable and Interminable," in *Standard Edition of Complete Psychological Works,* vol. 23, London: Hogarth Press, 1964, pp. 209–253.
42. Knight, R. P.: Evaluation of Results of Psychoanalytic Therapy, *Amer. J. Psychiat.,* 98:434, 1941.
43. Ubell, E.: Psychiatric Treatment Results Are Measured, *New York Herald Tribune,* July 7, 1958.
44. Brody, M. W.: "Prognosis and Results of Psychoanalysis," in Nodine, J. H., and Moyer, J. H. (eds.): *Psychosomatic Medicine,* Philadelphia: Lea and Febiger, 1962, pp. 729–733.
45. Masserman, J. H.: "Etiology, Comparative Biodynamics, and Psychoanalytic Research," in Scher, J. M. (ed.): *Theories of the Mind,* New York: Free Press, 1962, pp. 15–64.
46. Heilbrunn, G.: Results with Psychoanalytic Therapy and Professional Commitment, *Amer. J. Psychother.,* 20:89, 1966.
47. Jacobson, E.: *Progressive Relaxation,* Chicago: University of Chicago Press, 1929.
48. Denker, P. G.: Results of Treatment of Psychoneuroses by General Practitioner, *N. Y. J. Med.,* 46:2164, 1946.
49. Neustatter, W. L.: Results of 50 Cases Treated by Psychotherapy, *Lancet,* 1:796, 1935.
50. Miles, H. H. W., Barrabee, E. L., and Finesinger, J. E.: Evaluation of Psychotherapy, *Psychosom. Med.,* 13:83, 1951.
51. Fiedler, F. E.: Comparison of Therapeutic Relationships in Psychoanalytic, Nondirective and Adlerian Therapy, *J. Consult. Psychol.,* 14:436, 1950.
52. Appel, K. E., Lhamon, W. T., Meyers, J. M., and Harvey, W. A.: "Long Term Psychotherapy," Proceedings of the Association for Research in Nervous and Mental Diseases, in *Psychiatric Treatment,* Baltimore: Williams and Wilkins, 1953, pp. 21–34.
53. Alexander, F.: "Evaluation of Psychotherapy," in Hoch, P. H., and Zubin, J: *Evaluation of Psychiatric Treatment,* New York: Grune & Stratton, 1964.
54. Glover, E.: Research Methods in Psychoanalysis, *Int. J. Psychoanal.,* 33:403, 1952.
55. Stevenson, I.: Processes of "Spontaneous" Recovery from Psychoneuroses, *Amer. J. Psychiat.,* 117:1057, 1961.
56. Eysenck, H. J.: Effects of Psychotherapy, *Int. J. Psychiat.,* 1:97, 1965.
57. Wolpe, J.: *Psychotherapy by Reciprocal Inhibition,* Stanford: Stanford University Press, 1958.
58. Lazarus, A. A.: Results of Behavior Therapy in 126 Cases of Severe Neurosis, *Behav. Res. Ther.,* 1:69, 1963.

59. Wolpe, J.: Prognosis of Unpsychoanalyzed Recovery from Neuroses, *Amer. J. Psychiat.*, 118:35, 1961.
60. Marks, I. M., and Gelder, M. G.: Controlled Retrospective Study of Behavior Therapy in Phobic Patients, *Brit. J. Psychiat.*, 11:561, 1965.
61. Ackerknecht, E. H.: *Short History of Psychiatry*, New York: Hafner, 1959.
62. Frank, J. D.: *Persuasion and Healing*, Baltimore: Johns Hopkins Press, 1961.
63. (a) Frank, J. D., Gliedman, L. H., Imber, S. D., Stone, A. R., Nash, E. H.: Patients' Expectancies and Relearning as Factors Determining Improvement in Psychotherapy, *Amer. J. Psychiat.*, 115:961, 1959.
   (b) Whitehorn, J. D., and Betz, B. J.: Further Studies of the Doctor as Crucial Variable in Outcome of Treatment with Schizophrenic Patients, *Amer. J. Psychiat.*, 117:215, 1960.
64. Wright, R.: *Hydrotherapy in Hospitals for Mental Diseases*, Boston: Tudor Press, 1932.
65. Young, G.: *Treatise on Opium Founded Upon Practical Observations*, London: Millar, 1753.
66. Brandeth, J. P.: *Medical Commentaries for Year MDCCXCI*, Edinburgh, 1792.
67. Bucknill, J. D., and Tuke, D. H.: *Manual of Psychological Medicine*, Philadelphia: Blanchard and Lea, 1858.
68. Carlson, E. T., and Simpson, M. M.: Opium as a Tranquilizer, *Amer. J. Psychiat.*, 120:112, 1963.
69. Clarke, E. H.: *Physiological and Therapeutical Action of the Bromide of Potassium and Bromide of Ammonium*, Boston: James Campbell, 1872.
70. Liebreich, O.: Das Chloral, ein neues Hypnoticum and Anästheticum, *Wien. Med. Wschr.*, 19:1087, 1869.
71. Weatherill, H. M.: Modern Hypnotics, *Amer. J. Insanity*, 46:28, 1888–1889.
72. Fisher, E., and von Mering, J.: Ueber eine neue Classe von Schlafmitteln, *Ther. Gegenw.*, 44:97, 1903.
73. Murray, G. R.: Note on Treatment of Myxoedema by Hypodermic Injections of Extract of Thyroid Gland of Sheep, *Brit. Med. J.*, 2:796, 1891.
74. Goldberger, J.: Prevention and Treatment of Pellagra, *Public Health Serv. Rep.*, 29:2821, 1914.
75. Elvehjem, C. A.: Isolation and Identification of Anti-Black Tongue Factor, *J. Biol. Chem.*, 123–137, 1938.
76. Wagner von Jauregg, J.: Ueber die Einwirkung fieberhafter Erkrankungen auf Psychosen, *Jb. Psychiat.*, 7:94, 1887.
77. Wagner von Jauregg, J.: Ueber die Einwirkung der Malaria aud die Progressive Paralyse, *Psychiat. Neurol. Wschr.*, 20:132, 1918–1919.
78. Fleming, A.: On Antibacterial Action of Cultures of Penicillium, *Brit. J. Exp. Path.*, 10:226, 1929.
79. Mahoney, J. F.: Penicillin Treatment of Early Syphilis, *Amer. J. Public Health*, 33:1387, 1943.
80. Sakel, M. J.: Schizophreniebehandlung mittels Insulin-Hypoglykämie sowie Hypoglykämischer Schocks, *Wien. Med. Wschr.*, 84:1211, 1934.
81. Dussik, K. T., and Sakel, M. J.: Ergenbnisse der Hypoglykämieschokbehandling der Schizophrenie, *Z. Ges. Neurol. Psychiat.*, 155, 1936.
82. Sakel, M. J.: "Classical Sakel Shock Treatment: A Reappraisal," in Sackler, A. M., et al (eds.): *Great Physiodynamic Therapies in Psychiatry*, New York: Paul B. Hoeber, 1956.

83. Ross, J. R., and Malzberg, G.: Review of the Results of Pharmacological Shock Therapy and Metrazol Convulsive Therapy in New York State, *Amer. J. Psychiat.*, 96:297, 1939.
84. Rennie, T. A. C.: Prognosis in Manic-Depressive and Schizophrenic Conditions Following Shock Treatment, *Psychiat. Quart.*, 17:642, 1943.
85. Bond, E. D., and Rivers, T. D.: Insulin Shock Therapy After Seven Years, *Amer. J. Psychiat.*, 101:62, 1944.
86. Gottlieb, J. S., and Huston, P. E.: Treatment of Schizophrenia, Comparison of Three Methods: Brief Psychotherapy, Insulin Coma and Electric Shock, *J. Nerv. Ment. Dis.*, 113:211, 1951.
87. Ackner, B., Harris, A., and Oldham, A. J.: Insulin Treatment of Schizophrenia: A Controlled Study, *Lancet*, 1:607, 1957.
88. Bond, E. D.: Results of Treatment in Psychoses with Control Series, *Amer. J. Psychiat.*, 110:881, 1954.
89. West, F. H., Bond, E. D., Shurley, J. T., and Meyers, C. D.: Insulin Coma Therapy in Schizophrenia: Fourteen-Year Follow-Up Study, *Amer. J. Psychiat.*, 111:583, 1955.
90. Hoff, H.: *Wien. Med. Wschr.*, 110:756, 1960.
91. Meduna, L.: Versuche uber die biologische Beeinflussing des Ablaufes der Schizophrenie: I. Campher-und Cardiazol Krampfe, *Z. Ges. Neurol. Psychiat.*, 152:235, 1935.
92. Cited by Meduna, L.: "Convulsive Treatment: A Reappraisal," in Sackler, A. M., et al (eds.): *Great Physiodynamic Therapies in Psychiatry*, New York: Paul B. Hoeber, 1956.
93. Cook, L. C.: "Convulsion Therapy," in Fleming, G. (ed.): *Recent Progress in Psychiatry*, London: Churchill, 1944.
94. Cerletti, U., and Bini, L.: Un nuovo metodo di shockterapia: "L'elettroshock," *Boll. e Atti della R. Accad. Med. di Roma*, 64:136–138, 1938.
95. Kalinowsky, L. B., and Worthing, H. J.: Results with Electric Convulsive Treatment in 200 Cases of Schizophrenia, *Psychiat. Quart.*, 17:144, 1943.
96. Hoch, P. H.: Progress in Psychiatric Therapies, *Amer. J. Quart. Psychiat.*, 112:241, 1955.
97. Verstraeten, P.: Thérapeutique convulsiante de la psychose maniaco-depressive, *Ann. Medicopsychol.*, 95 II:654, 1937.
98. Huston, P., and Locher, L. M.: Involutional Psychosis: Course When Untreated and When Treated with Electric Shock, *Arch. Neurol. Psychiat.*, 59:385, 1948.
99. Huston, P., and Locher, L. M.: Manic-Depressive Psychosis: Course When Untreated and Treated with Electric Shock, *Arch. Neurol. and Psychiat.*, 60:37, 1948.
100. Egas Moniz, A. C.: *Tentatives opérations dans le traitment de certaines psychoses*, Paris: Masson, 1936.
101. Freeman, W., and Watts, J. W.: *Psychosurgery*, Springfield, Ill.: Charles C. Thomas, 1942.
102. Freeman, W.: Prefrontal Lobotomy, 1936–1956: Follow-Up Study of 3000 Patients from One to Twenty Years, *Amer. J. Psychiat.*, 113:817, 1957.
103. Kalinowsky, L. B., and Hoch, P. H.: *Somatic Treatments in Psychiatry*, New York: Grune & Stratton, 1961.
104. Laborit, H.: Hibernation artificielle, *Acta Anesth. Belg.*, 2:710, 1951.
105. Delay, J., and Deniker, P.: Chlorpromazine and Neuroleptic Treatments in Psychiatry, *J. Clin. Exp. Psychopath.*, 17:19–24, 1956.

106. Kinross-Wright, V.: Chlorpromazine Treatment of Mental Disorders, *Amer. J. Psychiat.*, 111:907, 1955.
107. Borsa, J. A., and Kline, N. S.: Use of Reserpine in Disturbed Psychotic Patients, *Amer. J. Psychiat.*, 112:684, 1956.
108. Malitz, S., Hoch, P. H., and Lesse, S.: Two Year Evaluation of Chlorpromazine in Clinical Research and Practice, *Amer. J. Psychiat.*, 113:540, 1956.
109. Winkleman, N. W.: Appraisal of Chlorpromazine, *Amer. J. Psychiat.*, 113:961, 1957.
110. Denker, H. C. B., and Bird, E. G.: Chlorpromazine in Treatment of Mental Illness, *Amer. J. Psychiat.*, 113:972, 1957.
111. Winkleman, N. W.: Clinical and Socio-Cultural Study of 200 Psychiatric Patients Started on Chlorpromazine 10½ Years Ago, *Amer. J. Psychiat.*, 120:861, 1964.
112. Brill, H., and Patton, R. E.: Clinical-Statistical Analysis of Population Changes in New York State Mental Hospitals Since Introduction of Psychotropic Drugs, *Amer. J. Psychiat.*, 119:20, 1962.
113. Robin, A. A.: Effect of Tranquilizers on Some Aspects of Treatment of Long Stay Patients, *Amer. J. Psychiat.*, 119:1076, 1963.
114. Loomer, H. P., Saunders, J. C., and Kline, N. S.: Clinical and Pharmacodynamic Evaluation of Iproniazid as Psychic Energizer, *Res. Rep. Amer. Psychiat. Assoc.*, 8:129, 1957.
115. Lehman, H. E., Cahn, C. H., and Verteuil, R. L.: Treatment of Depressive Conditions with Imipramine, *Canad. Psychiat. Assoc. J.*, 3:155, 1958.
116. Cole, J. O.: Therapeutic Efficacy of Antidepressant Drugs, *JAMA*, 190:448, 1964.
117. Greenblatt, M., Grosser, G. A., and Wechsler, H.: Comparative Study of Selected Antidepressant Medications and EST, *Amer. J. Psychiat.*, 119:144, 1962.
118. Schou, M., Juel-Neilson, N., Strömgren, E. and Voldby, H.: Treatment of Manic Psychoses by Administration of Lithium Salts, *J. Neurol. Neurosurg. Psychiat.*, 17:250, 1954.
119. Wortis, J.: Review of Psychiatric Progress: Physiological Treatment, *Amer. J. Psychiat.*, 117:595, 1961.
120. Cole, J. O., et al: Phenothiazine Treatment in Acute Schizophrenia, *Arch. Gen. Psychiat.*, 10:246, 1964.
121. Elkes, J.: American College of Neuropsychopharmacology—A Note on Its History and Hopes for Future, *Bull. Am. Coll. Neuropsychopharm.*, vol. 1, no. 5, May 1963.
122. Hobbs, N.: Mental Health's Third Revolution, *Am. J. Orthopsychiat.*, 34:822, 1964.
123. Dunham, H. W.: Community Psychiatry—Newest Therapeutic Bandwagon, *Arch. Gen. Psychiat.*, 12:303, 1965.
124. Burrows, G. M.: *Commentaries on Causes, Forms, Symptoms and Treatment, Moral and Medical, of Insanity*, London: Thomas and George Underwood, 1828.
125. Brigham, A.: *Remarks Upon Influence of Mental Cultivation Upon Health*, Hartford: Huntington, 1832.
126. Channing, W.: Some Remarks on Address Delivered to American Medico-Psychological Association by S. Weir Mitchell, MD, May 16, 1894, *Amer. J. Insanity*, 51:171, 1894–1895.
127. *Action for Mental Health: Final Report of Joint Commission on Mental Illness and Health*, New York: Basic Books, 1961.

128. Cumming, J., and Cumming, E.: *Ego and Milieu: Theory and Practice of Environmental Therapy,* New York: Atherton Press, 1962.
129. Greenberg, E. M. (ed.): Evaluating Effectiveness of Mental Health Services, *Milbank Mem. Fund Quart.,* vol. 44, no. 1, January 1966.
130. Binner, P. R.: Studies of the Fort Logan Program, in Reference 122, pp. 320–336.

PRESENT DIRECTIONS
AND EVOLVING PROGRAMS
IN PSYCHIATRIC CARE

2

Psychopharmacology in the Large Mental Hospital in Transition*

by MILTON GREENBLATT
and MYRON R. SHARAF

Greenblatt and Sharaf delineate from their own experience the manner in which the mental hospital evolved from its previous custodial state to a hospital in transition. They describe the development and strategies of new patterns of psychiatric care in the hospital, clinic, home, and community—patterns that involve a sophisticated synthesis of social, psychologic, biologic, and psychopharmacologic practice. Many of the contributions described are derived from Greenblatt's own outstanding clinical, experimental, and administrative investigations. As Commissioner of Mental Health, the Commonwealth of Massachusetts, Dr. Greenblatt seeks to open new avenues for helping the mentally ill. This chapter reveals the authors' firm knowledge and vision as contemporary and future psychiatry is set forth.

During the last few years the large mental hospital has been undergoing rapid changes from custodial institution to therapeutic community and from therapeutic community to community mental health center. During this period we have also seen the rapid

* Presented at the Annual Meeting of the American College of Neuropsychopharmacology, Puerto Rico, December 1966.

expanding of psychopharmacology as a leading therapeutic modality, a nexus of multidisciplinary research activity, and an area for legitimate education of mental health professionals. It is interesting to view the changes in the psychopharmacologic scene against the dramatic developments occurring along the entire mental health front. The attempt here is to sketch a rough picture of the relationships in four areas: (a) use of drugs in the inpatient service; (b) outpatient and aftercare services; (c) hospital extension services or home treatment; (d) use of drugs by general practitioners coping with emotional disorders in the community.

As superintendent of a large mental hospital, one is in a strategic position to effect change, to coordinate and integrate therapeutic activities, and to instigate studies thereof. Boston State Hospital, like many in the nation, has experienced an almost explosive development of programs and services within a few short years. These include a halfway house, day center, night center, day school for the retarded, adolescent service, alcohol service, rehabilitation service, screening unit, child psychiatry program, home treatment service, addiction center, general practitioner and family care programs, as well as dramatic expansion of training and research. As in many other state hospitals in the nation, there has been a sharp reduction in the inpatient census, as shown by Figure 1.

Fig. 1

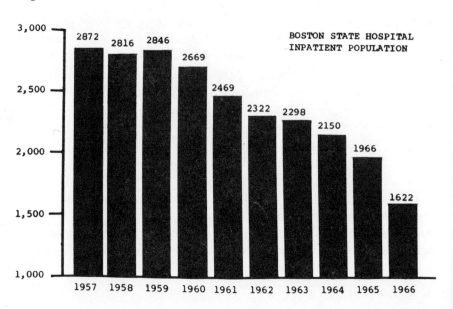

BOSTON STATE HOSPITAL
INPATIENT POPULATION

3,000 — 2872 2816 2846
2669
2,500 — 2469
2322 2298
2150
2,000 — 1966
1622
1,500 —
1,000 —
        1957 1958 1959 1960 1961 1962 1963 1964 1965 1966

Overcrowding has been relieved; in fact, we have been able to make six buildings available, converting three of these to a retardation center, adolescent school plus recreation hall, and night hospital, respectively. The remaining three, awaiting demolition, are unfit for human habitation. Many have claimed that the downward trend in residential patients is due to the psychopharmacologic revolution. Our wiser colleagues know, however, that this trend was establishing itself in some vanguard hospitals before the advent of the tranquilizer era, through the judicious introduction of social psychiatric methods. Pharmaceuticals, nevertheless, did play a paramount if not an exclusive role in the transition.

Intersecting the downward trend of inpatient population is an almost opposite rise in admissions, which have doubled in the last eight to ten years. A vast increase in patients treated in transitional facilities or aftercare services shows less overall time spent in the hospital, though the total number of patients looked after is greater than before. One could dwell at length on the fascinating subject of institutional change, but we will limit our discourse mainly to the area of psychopharmacology.

I DRUGS AND INPATIENTS

Table 1 shows the astonishing rise of psychopharmacotherapy at Boston State Hospital over ten years, expressed as "pills pushed" and counted by the pharmacist.[1] Note a 15-fold rise from 1955 to 1965 for inpatients. The table further indicates that the number of

TABLE 1

**Boston State Hospital
Psychopharmaceuticals
Total Tablets Dispensed**

1965	1960	1955
1,675,190	854,109	113,503
(44,677)*	(9,238)*	(–0–)

* Tablets Dispensed for Outpatient Use During One Month of the Year.

tablets dispensed in the Out Patient Department (OPD) has shown a dramatic rise from zero in 1955 to 44,677 in 1965. This is based on a one-month figure of drugs dispensed. The annual picture may be assumed to be about 12 times the figure in parentheses. The table also indicates that the proportion of drugs prescribed for outpatients is rising relative to that prescribed for inpatients. For 1960 the outpatient prescriptions were 12.9% of the total, and in 1965, 32% of the total. Obviously, psychopharmacotherapy has become big business within a few short years; yet many claim that neither the administration of drugs nor the teaching of psychopharmacology has kept pace with the clinical developments in other treatment modalities.

TABLE 2

Boston State Hospital
Psychopharmaceuticals

		TOTAL TABLETS DISPENSED		
		1965	1960	1955
Major Tranquilizers				
chlorpromazine	THORAZINE	455,413	131,945	102,978
trifluoperazine	STELAZINE	312,497	138,327	
thioridazine	MELLARIL	190,273	161,931	
perphenazine	TRILAFON	90,305		
carphenazine maleate	PROKETAZINE	32,770		
chlorprothixine	TARACTAN	31,800		
prochlorperazine	COMPAZINE	23,988		
fluphenazine HCl	PROLIXIN	17,338		
promazine	SPARINE	10,906		
triflupromazine	VESPRIN		13,984	
Minor Tranquilizers				
chlordiazepoxide	LIBRIUM	90,828		
meprobamate	MILTOWN, EQUANIL	24,261	70,432	
diazepam	VALIUM	11,496		
mepazine	PACATAL		2,450	
reserpine		348	10,110	10,525
Antidepressants				
imipramine	TOFRĀNIL	248,562	107,771	
amitriptyline HCl	ELAVIL	122,888		
phenelzine sulfate	NARDIL	1,355	13,625	
meprobamate and benactyzine HCl	DEPROL	962	2,111	

Table 2 shows drugs used in the ten-year span, broken down into classes: major tranquilizers, minor tranquilizers, and antidepressants.[1] Chlorpromazine (Thorazine), trifluoperazine (Stelazine), and thioridazine (Mellaril) today lead the pack, with a variety of lesser competitors crowding the field; triflupromazine (Vesprin), which had a short life around 1960, has all but disappeared. Among minor tranquilizers, chlordiazepoxide HCI (Librium) now leads the field; meprobamate (Miltown or Equanil) has declined in popularity, and reserpine has essentially disappeared. Imipramine (Tofrānil) and amitriptyline HCl (Elavil) are most prescribed among the antidepressants; phenelzine sulphate (Nardil) and meprobamate and benactyzine HCl (Deprol) have declined.

Taking the shorter time span, we are fortunate to be able to compare the years 1963 and 1965 in the month of October, through the kindness of Schulberg and Notman.[2] Even during this brief period there have been dramatic shifts. We limited ourselves to drugs used on ten or more patients (out of approximately 2,300 in 1963 and 1,900 in 1965). Table 3 presents both numbers and percentages of patients taking various drugs.

TABLE 3

Major Tranquilizers Administered to Inpatients*

		October 1963		October 1965	
		Number	%	Number	%
chlorpromazine	THORAZINE	353	41.52	332	37.77
trifluoperazine	STELAZINE	251	29.52	167	19.00
thioridazine	MELLARIL	26	3.05	124	14.11
perphenazine	TRILAFON	——	——	97	11.04
trifluoperazine &	STELAZINE &				
chlorpromazine	THORAZINE	30	3.52	63	7.17
chlorprothixine	TARACTAN	28	3.29	22	2.50
carphenazine maleate	PROKETAZINE	49	5.76	14	1.59
prochlorperazine	COMPAZINE	52	6.11	11	1.25
fluphenazine HC1	PROLIXIN	25	2.94	8	0.91
promazine	SPARINE	34	4.00	6	0.68

* From Schulberg and Notman with permission.

During the two years we note a definite drop in the use of chlorpromazine (41.5% to 37.8%); trifluoperazine (29.5% to 19.0%); carphenazine maleate (Proketazine) (5.8% to 1.6%); prochlorperazine (Compazine) (6.1% to 1.2%); and promazine (Sparine) (4.0% to 1%). On the other hand, there is a sharp rise in the use of perphenazine (Trilafon) (from 0 to 11.0%), thioridazine (3.0% to 14.1%), and trifluoperazine-chlorpromazine combination (3.5% to 7.1%). It is an interesting fact that the overall absolute number of inpatients on drugs in the two years is only slightly increased, but since the inpatient population has decreased dramatically a substantial percentage rise in the use of psychopharmacotherapy appears.

TABLE 4
Minor Tranquilizers Administered to Inpatients*

		October 1963		October 1965	
		Number	%	Number	%
chlordiazepoxide	LIBRIUM	14	20.00	23	41.81
phenobarbital		37	52.85	12	21.81
diazepam	VALIUM	—	——	8	14.54
oxazepam	SERAX	—	——	7	12.72
meprobamate	EQUANIL, MILTOWN	19	27.13	4	7.25

* From Schulberg and Notman with permission.

Again, from Schulberg and Notman's data on minor tranquilizers, we learn in Table 4 that chlordiazepoxide has advanced from 20% to 41.8%; diazepam (Valium) from 0 to 14.5%; oxazepam (Serax) from 0 to 12.7%. Meprobamate, however, shows a decline from 27.1% to 7.2%, and phenobarbital from 52.9% to 21.8%. The overall use of minor tranquilizers is not great for a hospital such as ours, with a significant decrease noted for the two periods (70 patients versus 54 patients in the two years). The declining use of minor tranquilizers may be related to the treatment of many of the milder disturbances—formerly admitted into the hospital—by practitioners outside or by members of our aftercare team in a OPD relationship.

As to antidepressants, Table 5 indicates that imipramine has increased from 38.2% to 65.1%, while amitriptyline HCl decreased from 57.4% to 27.7%. A very considerable increase in the number of patients receiving antidepressants (47 to 155) may reflect drug-specific research in this field at Boston State Hospital.

How does the overall use of psychopharmacotherapy compare with other treatment modalities? As Table 6 indicates,* again com-

* Definition of therapies: *Verbal treatments* include individual psychotherapy, group psychotherapy, individual counseling, group counseling, and casework. *Somatic treatments* include electric shock, major tranquilizers, minor tranquilizers, and anti-depressants. *Activity treatments* include work therapy, occupational and activity therapy, and recreational therapy.

TABLE 5

Antidepressants Administered to Inpatients*

		October 1963		October 1965	
		Number	%	Number	%
imipramine	TOFRĀNIL	18	38.29	101	65.16
amitriptyline HCl	ELAVIL	27	57.44	43	27.74
nortriptyline HCl	AVENTYL	—	——	5	3.22
desipramine HCl	PERTOFRANE, NORPRAMIN	—	——	4	2.57
isocarboxazid	MARPLAN	—	——	2	1.29
methylphenidate HCl	RITALIN	2	4.25	1	0.64
meprobamate and benactyzine HCl	DEPROL	—	——	1	0.64

* From Schulberg and Notman with permission.

TABLE 6

Types of Therapies Received by Inpatients*

	October 1963		October 1965	
	Number	%	Number	%
Somatic Alone	541	24.04	648	34.47
Somatic and Activity	227	10.13	260	13.83
Verbal and Somatic	96	4.27	202	10.74
Verbal, Activity, and Somatic	155	6.89	179	9.52
Activity Alone	243	10.80	112	5.96
Verbal Alone	89	3.96	91	4.84
Verbal and Activity	69	3.07	49	2.61
None	829	36.84	339	18.03
Total	2,249	100.00	1,880	100.00

* From Schulberg and Notman with permission.

paring 1963 and 1965, there has been a rise in "somatic therapy alone"—including a small amount of electroconvulsive therapy (ECT)—during two years from 24% to 34.5%. There has also been a rise in combined "somatic and other therapies" from 45.3% to 68.6% (sum of lines 1, 2, 3, and 4 of the Table). This increase in the use of somatic treatments has not been accompanied by a decline in verbal therapies; on the contrary, a rise is shown in the latter from 18.2% to 27.7%. I suppose our proudest figure would be the decline in patients receiving *no therapy*, from 36.8% to 18.0%.

Summarizing, therapy in general is more active; fewer patients are neglected. A tendency toward polypharmacy is noted; perphenazine is making inroads on chlorpromazine and trifluoperazine; the use of thioridazine is increasing (perhaps because of publication of long-term untoward side effects with chlorpromazine and trifluoperazine); phenobarbital is giving way to antidepressants; the switch from amitriptyline HCl to imipramine is of interest and may be artifactual (result of research); chlordiazepoxide overshadows promazine (with use in alcoholism rising); and there is a noteworthy drop of the number of patients on minor tranquilizers.

II   DRUGS AND OUTPATIENTS

The most dramatic change occurs in the amount of psychopharmacotherapy administered to outpatients. An outpatient is defined simply as anyone not on 24-hour status in the hospital, and includes, therefore, day patients, halfway house residents, night patients, regular outpatients, aftercare patients, apartment dwellers, family care patients, and so on.

TABLE 7

Boston State Hospital
Pharmacy Department

Calendar Year	Number of OPD Prescriptions
1957 and all previous years	0
1958	658
1959	2,100
1960	2,731
1961	4,601
1962	8,506
1963	11,261
1964	16,702
1965	20,353
1966	over 24,000 estimated

Table 7 shows that awesome year-by-year increase in medication given to outpatients.[1] Prior to 1957 and during all previous years in the memory of our pharmacist, who has served for 36 years, no prescriptions were given to patients defined as outpatients. In 1950 the Briggs Outpatient Clinic was established at Boston State Hospital, and rapidly thereafter a number of the transitional facilities mentioned above. As these were set up, the staff in all buildings ventured to discharge patients more readily and to maintain after-care services connected with their buildings in which all echelons of staff participated. During this time the hospital recognized its responsibility to provide drugs for indigent outpatients; the budget was increased proportionately. This table makes obvious the great shift in care from hospital to community within the last decade. For the convenience of patients on psychopharmacotherapy and for greater efficiency, we plan a second OPD pharmacy, to be established in the near future in the New Barton Mental Health Center. This Center, closer to the city traffic lines, will relieve the currently overburdened pharmacy staff in our Medical-Surgical Building.

III DRUGS AND HOME TREATMENT

In 1957 the pioneering Home Treatment Service was established at Boston State Hospital by Drs. Barton, Mann, and Friedman,[3] serving the Dorchester area's 190,000 people. Based in the hospital, the psychiatric team goes out into the community to provide evaluation and treatment for those patients suffering from severe mental illness who for some reason or other cannot obtain adequate help from existing facilities. By bringing help to patients and families when they need it and where they need it, the following multiple advantages accrue: (1) more realistic appraisal of both the home situation and the family interaction; (2) mobilization of community resources in the patient's behalf; (3) prevention of hospitalization in at least 50% of those so destined, thus eliminating the stigma of mental hospitalization and maintaining the patient's ties to family, community, and job. In those cases where hospitalization is indicated, the home visit also is a valuable adjunct in preparing the patient for admission.

Pharmacotherapy is one of the basic treatment tools employed by Home Treatment Service. For example,[4] of 119 psychotic patients treated in the sixteen months beginning November 1962, all but four received psychopharmaceuticals. In 63 cases phenothiazines were used; in 23 cases, antidepressants; in 21, a combination of antidepressants and phenothiazines; and in 8 cases other drugs were used.

The Service's psychiatrists believe in the efficacy of these drugs in the treatment of the very sick patients referred to them. However, beyond this there are other factors. For example: (a) the family often need tangible evidence that something is being done for the patient and are reassured by prescription of drugs; (b) the family doctor, whose treatment inclination is basically somatic, can relate more easily to the patient and the psychiatric team (prescription of drugs also gives the Home Treatment Service a focus of consultation with the general practitioner); (c) lastly, psychopharmacotherapy counters the anxiety of the Home Treatment team itself about treating and maintaining sick patients in the community.

The Home Treatment Service places great reliance on teamwork and on the nurse or psychiatric social worker as an extension of the psychiatrist. The nurse is often the prime therapeutic agent, visiting the patient on a regular basis, guiding individual and family therapy, and monitoring psychopharmacotherapy, reporting back reactions, side effects, and general progress. Discussions with the psychiatrist take place during the thrice-weekly staff conferences, or during the once-weekly individual supervision in which the nurse's caseload is discussed. The important potential of the nurse in home treatment and the dramatic changes in her role were not foreseen when the Home Treatment Service was inaugurated in 1957.

IV   DRUGS AND THE GENERAL PRACTITIONER

In connection with studies in the Home Treatment Service, in 1962 the general practitioners throughout the Dorchester area were queried as to their use of psychopharmaceuticals with the severely ill.[5] Of 87 whose responses were analyzed, 43 were then using chlorpromazine and prochlorperazine exclusively; 22 used prochlorperazine, and 9 chlorpromazine only; 13 did not use either drug. In general, dosage level corresponded to minimal levels recommended by the highly conservative *Physicians' Desk Reference* (*PDR*). Perhaps this conservatism was responsible for prochlorperazine's being considered ineffective. Other drugs in popular use at that time included meprobamate, chlordiazepoxide, barbiturates, imipramine, amitriptyline HCl, trifluoperazine, meprobamate and benactyzine, dextroamphetamine sulphate and amobarbital, and thioridazine.

Information gathered on the general practitioner's use of particular drugs in the treatment of anxiety and depression showed that antidepressants were used to treat anxiety as well as depression, and tranquilizers to treat depression as well as anxiety. If there is surprise at this finding, an explanation can be found in the fact that complex syndromes often confront the general practitioner, who may not have psychiatric expertise in psychopharmacology, and also that the indications for the use of these drugs remain far from being fully clarified.

When drugs were ineffective, the general practitioner changed the drug rather than the dose. When a drug proved ineffective, he also often referred the patient to a psychiatrist.

Weiner and LaPointe have instituted a project recently wherein general practitioners treat the seriously ill in the wards of our Boston State Hospital, Dorchester Unit, in collaboration with the psychiatrist and other members of the mental health team.[6,7] In addition, the ill may receive consultation on request before referral as well as during aftercare. Many of these patients, whether hospitalized or not, are presented at staff conferences where the group of practitioners participate in collaboration with the other professionals. In addition, regular ongoing seminars in psychiatry are held for the practitioners.

Although this project is of recent date, it is obvious that general practitioners seem more comfortable with mentally ill patients and with mental health professionals, thus lending them much more confidence in their psychopharmacology.

V   EDUCATION AND RESEARCH

In any large mental hospital with a staff shortage, there is great concern about organization and effective supervision of drug therapy. Quality control entails not only a high degree of sophistication in prescription but effective monitoring and regular review. An all-too-familiar practice is to prescribe drugs without adequate checkup; thus, the patient may not be taking the drug at all, the dose may be unsatisfactory, or toxicity may go unrecognized.

The two important factors that contribute to inadequate education in drug therapy are *psychiatric treatment philosophy* and *institutional patterns* that diminish involvement in drug therapy.

Regarding *treatment philosophy*, it is well known that in many training centers Freudian or neo-Freudian philosophy has minimized or devalued the significance of other modes of treatment. Psychiatric residents trained largely in individual and group psychotherapy were less ready to understand the patient's total life in the hospital, including the meaning of his drug treatment. Often the resident tends to focus on negative aspects of psychopharmacotherapy; eg, it provided a "chemical straitjacket," which helped the overburdened ward staff to "control the patient."

Sharaf and Levinson[8] have delineated two orientations of psychiatric residents: a dominant "psychotherapeutic," which is more or less opposed to the use of somatic treatments, and an "eclectic" point of view, which is less exclusively committed to psychologic therapies. Klerman[9, 10] has indicated irrational factors both in the use *and* non-use of drugs. He has stressed the social psychology of the residency period, a time when the aspiring psychiatrist is deviating from his medical identity toward a new orientation of working *with* patients rather than doing things *to* them. It is not surprising that drug therapy is often considered as medical treatment and, therefore, devalued.

Nevertheless, drug use in almost all institutions is high. As noted above, 60% of patients at Boston State Hospital are receiving psychopharmacotherapy. A smaller nearby training institution reports 40% to 60% of their patients receiving drugs, usually in combination with other treatments.[10]

With the wide use of drug therapy available, what can be done to bring this treatment to stage center of resident education? At Boston State Hospital the upsurge of psychopharmacologic research and the appointment to the staff of career psychopharmacologists has been a spur to education in this field. Currently a somatic therapy seminar is given for residents and other staff members. More important, regular clinical case consultations are being developed for problems pertaining to drug therapy. In time we hope the resident will develop the kind of self-scrutiny relative to his use of drugs that now prevails in his study of psychotherapeutic maneuvers. He might thus find he has avoided using drug treatment chiefly because of a narcissistic desire to treat the patient by himself without psychopharmacologic assist; on the other hand, he might overmedicate a patient because of an inability to mobilize his psychologic resources in dealing with the patient and the staff.

Certain educational issues have been pinpointed more closely by Appleton and Chien.[11] Although they found that "psychotherapeutic" and "eclectic" residents prescribed drugs more or less equally, they noted that psychotherapeutically oriented residents were less inclined to change their original prescription and less inclined to continue patients on medication following discharge. In another study, Chien and Appleton[12] demonstrated that psychotherapeutic residents learned less about drug treatment over a six-month training period than did eclectic residents. In particular, the former lagged behind eclectic residents in learning about drug classification and side effects.

TABLE 8

Mean Score of Psychopharmacological Knowledge*

	Psychotherapeutic Resident	Eclectic Resident
Before Six-Month Training Period	63.5	not 68.7 sig.
After	79.5	87.0 sig.
	SIG.	SIG.

* From Chien and Appleton.

Concerning *institutional factors* that have prevented deeper involvement in drug treatment, perhaps the most glaring pertain to the lack of participation by patients themselves. Partly because psychiatrists and others are ambivalent about drug treatment, patients frequently are uninformed about the nature of the drugs they are receiving. Despite an excellent article by Havens[13] on the importance of patient responsibility in decision-making about drugs, such participation has been relatively rare. However, the growing interest in patient-staff meetings along "therapeutic community" lines may help to bring issues of drug treatment—along with other problems of individual and collective living in the hospital setting—to the forefront of shared discussion.

A change in administrative practice on one unit at Boston State Hospital, originally instigated to reduce the service load of psychiatric residents, gave two nurses administrative responsibility for their respective wards, with the resident psychiatrist serving as consultant. The nurse, like the resident, continued to function under supervision of the senior in charge of the service. The new arrangement made explicit what had formerly been implicit: that where residents covered several wards, their decisions usually tended to be official endorsement of those decisions already made by ward personnel.

One anticipated problem relative to this change concerned drug medication. What if the nurse and her consulting physician disagreed about medication? Who was the "boss"? In practice, however, there has been little disagreement. The nurse and resident amicably discuss medication, along with other issues, and in problem cases arrive at a "joint" decision. With this structural change in lines of authority there was an increased involvement on the part of the nurse in drug therapy. The nurse more carefully checked the effects of particular drugs and began to experiment with changes, especially in the direction of decreasing the dose for long-term cases. The patients were now *her* patients; she assumed the chief immediate responsibility for their care. This is an important instance of how a change in one aspect of a ward's organization can change, in an unanticipated fashion, the monitoring of drug treatment.

Another example of organizational change that may affect drug treatment is the unitization of the hospital, such as that which recently occurred at Boston State. Again, the chief reason for this change did not involve drug treatment per se. Rather, the central aims were to provide continuity of treatment for patients and closer ties with the community. Presently, each of four units at the hospital cares for both acute and long-term cases from a particular geographic area. Since transfer of case "failures" is not permissible, every case, acute or chronic, receives more intensive, responsible, and resourceful attention.

The rise in drug prescriptions for outpatients reflects our responsibility to treat indigent disturbed patients in the community. Within the community, lower-class patients perceive drugs as treatment for "bad nerves"; this they accept better than purely verbal therapy. A number of studies[14-16] stress the importance of meeting patients' expectations, be they for economic or medical aid, as a step in helping them with emotional problems. We must learn to understand how lower-class persons perceive us and what they want from us wherever drug treatment is used as a vehicle toward a deeper psychologic relationship.

Community psychiatry has implications for education about drug treatment at many levels. We noted earlier that the great majority of home treatment visits are made by nurses and social workers who assume the chief responsibility for monitoring pharmacologic treatment. It might also be stated that in drug therapy an increasing role is being played by the patient's family or his "foster family," as well as nursing-home personnel. The increased dispersion of patients among various care-giving groups in the community of course requires an accompanying dispersion of accurate knowledge about drugs.

The rapid changes in psychiatric practice suggested above heighten the importance of incorporating and integrating education about drugs into the resident's total clinical training program. We would urge continuing research on the personal-social characteristics of residents, as well as on the philosophic orientation in the training center, in those areas that promote or impede rational use of drugs. We would stress also that organizational changes of many types can effect patterns of drug treatment by personnel at many levels.

REFERENCES

1. Sicilano, J., Chief Pharmacist, Pharmacy Department, Boston State Hospital: Unpublished data and personal communication.
2. Schulberg, H. C., Notman, R., and Bookin, E.: Treatment Services at a Mental Hospital in Transition, *Amer. J. Psychiat.*, 124:506–513 (No. 4), 1967.
3. Weiner, L., Becker, A., and Friedman, T. T.: *Home Treatment: Spearhead of Community Psychiatry*, Boston State Hospital Monograph Series No. 1, Pittsburgh: University of Pittsburgh Press, 1967.
4. Meyer, E. R., Schiff, L. F., and Becker, A.: Home Treatment of Psychotic Patients: Analysis of 154 Cases, *Amer. J. Psychiat.*, 123:1430–38, 1967.
5. Weiner, L.: "General Medical Practitioner in Psychiatric Network," Chapter 10 in *Home Treatment: Spearhead of Community Psychiatry*, Boston State Hospital Monograph Series No. 1, Pittsburgh: University of Pittsburgh Press, 1967.
6. Weiner, L.: General Practitioner Psychiatric Consultation Program, *Psychiat. Op.*, 3:38–42 (No. 3), June 1966.
7. Weiner, L.: General Practitioner Psychiatric Consultation Program, *Psychiat. Op.*, 3:38–42 (No. 3), June 1966.
8. Sharaf, M. R., and Levinson, D. J.: "Patterns of Ideology and Role Definition Among Psychiatric Residents," in Greenblatt, M., Levinson, D. J., and Williams, R. H. (eds.): *The Patient and the Mental Hospital*, Glencoe, Ill.: Free Press, 1967, pp. 263–295.
9. Klerman, G. L., Sharaf, M. R., Holzman, M., and Levinson, D. J.: Sociopsychological Characteristics of Resident Psychiatrists and Their Use of Drug Therapy, *Amer. J. Psychiat.*, 111–117, 1960.
10. Klerman, G. L.: Teaching of Psychopharmacology in Psychiatric Residency, *Comp. Psychiat.*, 6:255–264 (No. 4), August 1965.
11. Chien, C., and Appleton, W. S.: Teaching of Psychopharmacology to First-Year Resident: Treatment Orientation and Learning, *Amer. J. Psychiat.* In press.
12. Appleton, W. S., and Chien, C.: Effect of Doctor's Attitude and Knowledge on His Use of Psychiatric Drugs, *J. Nerv. Ment. Dis.*, 145:284–291 (No. 4), 1967.
13. Havens, L. L.: Problems with Use of Drugs in Psychotherapy of Psychotic Patients, *Psychiatry*, 26:289–296, 1963.
14. Minuchin, S., Auerswald, E., King, C. H., and Rabinowitz, C.: Study and Treatment of Families That Produce Multiple Acting-out Boys, *Amer. J. Orthopsychiat.*, 34:125–133, 1964.
15. Brill, N. Q., and Storrow, H. A.: "Social Class and Psychiatric Treatment," in Riessman, F., Cohen, J., and Pearl, A. (eds.): *Mental Health of the Poor*, Glencoe, Ill.: Free Press, 1964, pp. 68–75.
16. Overall, B., and Aronson, H.: "Expectations of Psychotherapy in Patients of Lower Class," in *Mental Health of the Poor*, Glencoe, Ill.: Free Press, 1964, pp. 76–97.

3

Changing Patterns of Psychiatric Care and Its Effect on a Community: The Maryland Psychiatric Register*

by KURT GORWITZ, Sc.D.

Gorwitz briefly but importantly describes one of the most significant tools placed in our hands for use in scientific psychiatry: the Maryland Psychiatric Case Register, a major device that has already analyzed a number of specific research projects. The Register, the largest project of its type in the world, has served as a prototype for similar programs in other areas.

Gorwitz concludes, from the investigations done thus far, that this approach represents an evolving direction for practical and research uses. In this multidisciplinary milieu, biostatistic services are combined with new computer aids to program the anticipated costs of projects, the results of clinical trials, and the epidemiologic data. The many other questions and information obtainable from this project will continue to lend enlightenment concerning the ever-changing patterns of psychiatric care.

This chapter makes clear the widespread need for psychiatric case registers on a national scale and that an interchange of data is highly desirable for the gathering of new information and the projection of further needs.

In recent years, much emphasis has been placed on minimizing chronicity in the large state mental hospitals through the use of

---

* Presented at the Annual Meeting of the American College of Neuropsychopharmacology, Puerto Rico, December 1966.

intensive treatment methods along with early release. The extensive use of tranquilizing drugs during the last 15 years has, of course, been an important factor in reducing the need for hospitalization and rehospitalization and in aiding many mentally ill to function more adequately as family and community members.

Among the more obvious effects of this program has been the gradual reduction in the size of the state mental hospital patient populations. With this reduction there has been reflected a concomitant increase in the number of first admissions and readmissions; an increase in the number of patients treated in psychiatric inpatient and outpatient facilities; and a rapid and continuing expansion in the size of the cohort of former hospital patients functioning in the community. In Maryland's mental hospitals, a decrease in the average age of the patient population has been produced, as well as a decline in the number of beds occupied by psychotic patients, and a concurrent increase in the number of alcoholics and patients with psychoneurotic and personality disorders. With the establishment and expansion of community facilities and the coordination of services, we can expect this trend to continue and to influence profoundly the role, function, and program of the state hospital.

At the same time, some specific questions have been raised regarding these programs that have been difficult to answer. What is the relationship between length of hospitalization and probability of rehospitalization? What is the total number of bed days and hospital episodes per patient over an extended period of time? Has there been an actual decrease in length of hospitalization, or have we replaced one extended hospitalization with a series of short-term treatment episodes? Are these parameters related to identifiable and measurable patient characteristics, and how are they affected by supportive services provided for these individuals?

Heretofore we have been unable to answer questions of this type with precision because statistical programs traditionally have been limited to describing individual episodes of treatment. However, a means of follow-up is now provided by the Maryland Psychiatric Case Register, which sequentially links data for all psychiatric treatment services received by an individual.

The Register is a research program administered by the Maryland Department of Mental Hygiene in cooperation with the National Institute of Mental Health. In operation since July 1, 1961, it is the largest project of its type in the world, and serves as a prototype for similar programs planned in other areas. It is based on reports for each patient admission and termination routinely submitted by more than 150 public and private psychiatric inpatient and out-patient facilities, representing nearly all such services for Maryland residents. Reports from psychiatrists in private practice, although desirable, do not exist. This creates some bias in our data.

In the last seven years, more than 100,000 state residents (3% of the population) have been identified as receiving psychiatric care. For each of these, the total treatment record is linked and con-tinually updated on computer tape, thus providing the basic in-gredients for our research endeavors. This record is currently being increased by approximately 10,000 new individuals annually. Dur-ing the last year these facilities reported more than 35,000 admis-sions by some 25,000 individuals. The difference between the two numbers represents multiple services received by the same person in one or more facilities. At the time of admission, data are collected on such patient characteristics as psychiatric diagnosis, age, race, sex, education, religion, household composition, mobility, occupa-tion, and employment status. At the time of termination, basic data are collected regarding services received during the treatment epi-sode. Another report on the diagnosis is requested in order to provide data on any changes in diagnosis during treatment. Also, questions are asked as to whether or not the patient has made suicidal threats or suicidal gestures during the current period of illness, and whether or not he has a drinking problem. An additional query pertaining to drug abuse and drug dependency was added in October 1966. In those cases where there is an affirmative response, the facility is asked to identify the specific drug or drugs. A study analyzing these latter data is now in preparation. It is fully recog-nized that, relative to each of the above questions, there is probably considerable under-reporting; this, of course, presents a problem with no ready solution. A program is being developed to determine whether submitted data accurately reflect information contained in the records of the reporting facility. The problem thus exists that these records may be similarly incorrect or incomplete. However, these data can provide us with basic information when conserva-tively approached, and can serve as a base for further studies.

The original agreement in 1961 between the Department of Mental Hygiene and the National Institute of Mental Health pro-vided that the Maryland Register involve research only and that this information, therefore, would not be available for individual case finding or case management. This concept has since received legal reinforcement by a statute adopted in Maryland in 1963, which protects data of this type against subpoena and other court actions.

The findings of a number of studies have been presented at professional meetings and published in professional journals. A summary of these studies, together with some of their major findings, follows.

In May 1965, we published a paper that presented an analysis of one year of Register data.[1] During this one-year period (July 1, 1961 to June 30, 1962) psychotic disorders were the most frequently reported admissions diagnosed, representing 33.8% of inpatient and 22.6% of outpatient admissions. There has been somewhat of a change since that time, the number of admissions for alcoholism being presently substantially higher than those for psychotic disorders. Considerable information was presented regarding the relationship between number of admissions and number of persons admitted for various population segments, the paper showing that the frequency of multiple services varied by age, by race, by sex, and by place of residence. The occurrence of more than one episode of care was more frequent among white males between 18 and 64 years of age residing in a suburban county. During this year (1961–1962), 1.08% of Maryland's population were under care. Baltimore, however, which had experienced a substantial and selective in-and-out migration, had a one-year prevalence rate twice as high as the remainder of the state (1.62% compared with 0.86%). Further analysis, based on four years of Register data that is now available, is planned.

During November 1965, we presented a paper in which we studied patterns of retention, release, and rehospitalization for Maryland's three major state mental hospitals relative to patients classified by such factors as age, diagnosis, education, place of residence, type of commitment, marital status, race, and number of previous hospitalizations.[2] The study followed, until June 30, 1964, a cohort of admissions who had entered these three facilities between July 1961 and December 31, 1962. Thus, all cases were under observation from a minimum of 18 months to a maximum of 36 months. Prior to January 1963 these hospitals were segregated, with Negroes admitted to the one and white patients to the other two as well as to a third, smaller facility. One of the findings in this study was that for most types of patients the patterns of release and rehospitalization differed more between the two white hospitals than between the Negro hospital and the two white hospitals combined. In this instance, our conclusion was that hospital policy appeared to have more influence on these factors than race.

Three diagnostic groups were included in this study: (1) psychotics, (2) alcoholics, and (3) personality disorders. For each of these groups, the rate of rehospitalization was substantial (45%, 42%, and 32%, respectively, within 18 months after release), although most of those involved showed only a single additional treatment episode. The total days of care in this and subsequent hospitalizations nevertheless were fairly small (a median of 137, 54, and 54 bed days respectively, within 18 months after admission). That is, during this observation period, a newly admitted psychotic on the average spent one fourth of his time in the hospital and three fourths in the community. The other two cohorts were hospitalized for less than one tenth of this time, spending nine tenths in the community. In general, although those released earliest tended to be rehospitalized sooner than those who had remained longer, these differences disappeared with increasing time in the community. After one year, the cumulative probability of rehospitalization was virtually identical, regardless of length of original hospitalization, thus raising speculation as to the therapeutic value of extended inpatient care.

The never-married and those previously married had a greater rate of hospitalization and of clinic admission than those currently married; they also were retained longer in the hospital and had a substantially greater median total bed days. Among psychotic patients, however, those married were released earliest and were also rehospitalized sooner, indicating that family pressures might have been related to premature release. Our conclusion, based on the limited data available, indicates that, in general, patients who received post-hospital clinic care had a lower rate of rehospitalization than those who did not. Definite conclusions cannot be attained from this, however, until further analysis is made of the individuals who do, and do not, avail themselves of post-hospital clinic care, and of the type and extent of these services. Such an analysis is planned for the privately operated psychiatric hospitals, which, in Maryland, treat an appreciable number of patients. This also will offer a comparison with public facilities.

In a paper presented at a research conference in April 1966, we compared, for each of Baltimore's 159 census tracts, the rates of treated mental illness with rates of other public health factors, such as infant mortality, births without prenatal care, syphilis, and tuberculosis. Comparison rates also were made of certain socio-economic variables, such as overcrowding, children not living with both parents, family income, and the education of the head of household.[3] Our data showed a high degree of positive association between these three latter factors and those of public health. That is, the tracts with low socio-economic levels generally had rates indicating major public health problems and high rates of treated mental illnesses. The tracts with high socio-economic levels had low rates of these public health indices and also of mental illness. Although high admission rates for such diagnoses as schizophrenic reactions, alcoholism, mental retardation, and brain syndromes were found for tracts with low socio-economic levels, a reverse or negative relationship existed in admission rates for involutional and affective disorders, personality disorders, and psychoneuroses. Further studies related to this subject are planned, including a detailed field investigation of one or more of these tracts.

At this 1966 conference we also presented a paper based on an analysis of data concerning 14,420 individuals who were reported to be schizophrenic during one or more episodes of care between July 1961 and June 1964.[4] Of these, 7,321 were on facility rolls at the beginning of the study period; the remaining 7,099 subsequently were admitted for treatment. These 14,420 were equal to a rate of 4.4 per 1,000 Maryland residents. That is, at some time during this three-year period, one of every 225 of the state's residents was under treatment for schizophrenia in a psychiatric facility. Nonwhite rates were higher than comparable white rates for most age and sex groups, but the highest rate (more than 2% of the defined population) was for white males between the ages of 35 and 44 who were separated from their wives.

This study indicated that the diagnosis of schizophrenia is frequently not consistently made. Many of these patients during this three-year period showed a previous or subsequent treatment episode in which they received a different primary diagnosis. For example, 8.9% were also diagnosed as alcoholics,[5] and 6.9% were reported to be manic-depressive or otherwise psychotic. Nearly 95% of this cohort of schizophrenics had one or more hospital treatment episodes. The remaining 720 (or 5%) were reported to have received only outpatient services. Although this number might be expected to be reduced somewhat by the very young, by those who had been under observation for only a short period of time, or by those who had been hospitalized in other states or prior to the Register's establishment, it nevertheless represents a cohort of appreciable size. One of a series of future studies on schizophrenia will be concerned with this outpatient group and will examine the possible effect of drug therapy, other supportive services, family, and community influences in relation to length and severity of illness, and the patient's ability to function without hospital care. A series of comparable studies is also planned for other cohorts of patients, such as alcoholics and those with personality disorders.

One aspect of the Register's research deals with state residents who have received psychiatric services and are at risk of receiving additional care. Routine programs therefore have been developed for removing from the active Register files those individuals who have died or are known to have migrated from Maryland. This removal has provided extensive data on morbidity and mortality among the treated mentally ill, and a series of studies dealing with these factors is in preparation. Preliminary data, from our three-hospital study, indicated that mortality was proportionally substantially higher among the mentally ill than in the general population, these rates being high both during hospitalization and after release. Excessive rates were found for each of the three diagnostic groups included in this study, but they were particularly high for alcoholics, who showed rates up to nine times as high as comparable figures for the same age and sex group in the general population. Future studies will concentrate on comparisons of age-specific death rates for various cohorts of patients and the determination of life expectancy at various age levels. Comparisons will be made between those who have been hospitalized and those who received only outpatient services.[6] Also, these data will be related to comparable statistics for the general population of Maryland. Since the patient population is believed to be excessively concentrated among the lower socio-economic groups, where death rates may be higher than average, comparisons will be attempted not only with the general population but also with various population segments. Where differences are determined, detailed studies will be carried out to determine specific causes of death playing a role, together with an evaluation of socio-economic and cultural influences. Consideration also will be given to the interrelationship of physical and mental illnesses.

As mentioned earlier, Maryland's state-operated mental hospitals were segregated by race until January 1963. Thereafter, admissions were assigned to these hospitals on a regional basis. Since resident patients were not transferred as part of this desegregation, actual integration has not as yet been achieved. As of the date of this paper, Register data indicate that almost no Negroes are treated in private psychiatric hospitals or in the psychiatric wards of general hospitals. The former segregated state hospitals are still predominantly white and Negro as before. Therefore, six years after official desegregation, the majority of Negroes requiring hospitalization continue to be cared for in one facility. In Maryland, as in most other states, Negro admission rates to outpatient facilities are higher than comparable statistics for the white population. However, available Register data indicate that these figures do not necessarily reflect actual care provided. Our data indicate that Negro admissions were more concentrated in the Department's post-hospital clinics, and white patients were more widely distributed among all outpatient facilities. Further, Negro admissions were more likely to involve one or two treatment services, whereas white admissions more usually involved more extended episodes of care. Because of these apparent differences, one of our planned studies will investigate variations in psychiatric care provided for the white and nonwhite population segments, and will evaluate both patterns and extent of services.

Maryland's first comprehensive community mental health center opened in 1967 under the aegis of the Psychiatric Institute of the University of Maryland in cooperation with the Department of Mental Hygiene. Located just west of central Baltimore, it serves a catchment area with a population approaching 100,000. Register data indicate that this cohort includes a heavy concentration in the lower socio-economic levels who have higher-than-average admission rates to psychiatric inpatient and outpatient facilities.

The Register staff is developing a report evaluating data on trends in the extent, type, and patterns of psychiatric services that this population has received during recent years. A data-reporting system for the Center is now being established by a member of the Register staff, with financial support from a NIMH grant. It is hoped that this Center will provide a continuing series of statistics that will render some evaluation of its services as well as an indication of its effect in meeting previously unmet needs, and in changing patterns of existing care. It is fortunate that the Center staff will include a research director. This position has been set at a sufficiently high level so that we should be able to attract someone of superior caliber. It is expected that this person will work in close coordination with the Register staff in developing the analyses for this area and in the preparation of data for comparison with other comprehensive centers.

The preceding are designed to give some indication of the type of research possible through a psychiatric case register. It should be clear that such research will be based essentially on tabulations prepared from data available through information contained in the reports supplied by the participating facilities. However, a register potentially can serve a much broader purpose when used in conjunction with data available from other sources. Certainly, for example, data on the relationship of outpatient care and rehospitalization have very limited value without some evaluation of the extent and type of these services.

In addition, Maryland Register data can serve as an important tool in drug studies. Since the Register contains information on individuals seen in a large number of facilities, it can thus aid in the selection of a sample containing patients with some specified characteristics. Further, data can be provided on the subsequent treatment history of a cohort of patients who have received a particular type of therapy. One instance in which this was accomplished was following, after release from the Spring Grove State Hospital, a group of alcoholics who had been treated with LSD.

The establishment and maintenance of the Maryland Psychiatric Case Register is the result of the efforts of a number of people with diverse professional backgrounds. Its continuance is dependent on its effective employment as a research tool serving the community of mental health workers. In this, we invite your active participation and support.

REFERENCES

1. Bahn, A. K., et al: Services Received by Maryland Residents in Facilities Directed by a Psychiatrist, *Public Health Rep.*, May 1965.
2. Gorwitz, K., et al: Psychiatric Case Register Study of Release and Return Rates for State Mental Hospital Patients, *Public Health Rep.*, January 1967.
3. Klee, G. D., et al: Ecological Analysis of Diagnosed Mental Illness in Baltimore, presented at the American Psychiatric Association Regional Research Conference on Psychiatric Epidemiology and Mental Health Planning, Baltimore, Md., April 21, 1966.
4. Warthen, F. J., et al: Diagnosed Schizophrenia in Maryland, presented at

the American Psychiatric Association Regional Research Conference on Psychiatric Epidemiology and Mental Health Planning, Baltimore, Md., April 21, 1966.
5. Gorwitz, K., et al: Some Epidemiological Data on Alcoholism in Maryland, *Quart. J. Stud. Alcohol.*, April 1962.
6. Gorwitz, K., and Warthen, F. J.: On the Relationship of Desegregation of a State Mental Hospital System to Rates of Treated White and Non-White Mental Illness. In preparation.

4

Program Evaluation
and Planning in a New
Community Mental Health Service:
Two Years' Experience*

by ALVIN M. MESNIKOFF,

ROBERT L. SPITZER,

and JEAN ENDICOTT

With the aid of the New York State Psychiatric Institute, Psychiatric Division of Columbia University, and the Biometric Division of the New York State Mental Hygiene Department, the Washington Heights Community Mental Health Service has fully programmed and planned studies for a cohort of patients. These evaluations, performed with the most sophisticated biometric measures and mental health personnel, seek to answer questions of demographic and psychopathologic characteristics. The effectiveness of the mental health service for the total community is measured and the various treatment results studied. Only two years' experience is recorded, but the report of this collective experience, though only a relative beginning, will continue to prove helpful to future investigators as subsequent data is collected.

———————•◦◦◦◦•———————

* Adapted in part from the *Psychiatric Quarterly*, July 1967, and reprinted with permission. Supported by NIMH Grants 1 R20 MHO1957 and MHO8534.

I THE FIRST YEAR'S EXPERIENCE

The evaluation of a community mental health service can be separated into four questions: (1) What are the demographic and
psychopathologic characteristics of the population being served?
(2) To what extent are the mentally ill in this community actually
receiving services from the community facility? (3) To what extent
are the treatment programs designed to meet the needs of the
population? and (4) What are the long-term differential effects of
various treatment modalities?

This chapter describes a program evaluation of a new urban
community mental health service: the Washington Heights Community Service (WHCS) of the New York State Psychiatric Institute. During the first year of operation, procedures have been
established and data collected applicable to the first two questions
of evaluation. Relevant to the third question is the utilization of this
data to influence and shape the therapeutic program. In one sense,
the goal has been to develop a program rigid enough to act, yet
flexible enough to be subject to change.

The WHCS is the most recent development in the long-range plan
of the Department of Psychiatry, Columbia University, to center the
major portion of its clinical activity in the Washington Heights
Health District of New York City as a population resource to
support a variety of service, training, and research programs. During the ten years of operation of this project, other Washington
Heights mental health projects have studied the social history of the
area,[1] mental health problems in social agency case loads,[2] the
epidemiology of psychiatric emergencies in an urban health district,[3] the evolution of a community-based mental health orientation on a university psychiatric service,[4] and the attitudes of leaders
in an urban area.[5]

The Emergency Room and the Outpatient Department of the
Presbyterian Hospital have provided certain psychiatric services to
the local population, primarily initial evaluation and supportive and
drug therapy. However, though the Psychiatric Institute is a part of
the Columbia Presbyterian Medical Center, inpatient services were
not specifically available to this local population at the Psychiatric
Institute, since it was the policy of the Institute to admit selected
patients from the whole of New York State. This practice was
significantly changed in 1960 with the beginning of the Washington
Heights Community Care Program. The Program was directed

toward evaluating the outcome of treatment of a group of schizophrenic patients from this local area treated at the Psychiatric Institute, as compared with a group from the same district who received the traditional care: ie, hospitalization at Bellevue and Rockland State hospitals. Bellevue Hospital is the local city receiving hospital, whereas Rockland is the state hospital serving the Washington Heights district.

At the outset, care for patients in the first group was distributed among the several services at the Psychiatric Institute, constituting an additional responsibility superimposed on already existing programs. This approach was considered in respect to the new WHCS, and discarded. The Service was the first attempt, of course, to centralize patient care within the Psychiatric Institute in a specific service designed to meet the needs of the local population. The WHCS, made available through funding under the Hospital Improvement Program from the National Institute of Mental Health, was established with its own staff and physical plant, designed to provide a broad range of inpatient, partial hospitalization, and follow-up outpatient treatment.

The catchment area for the WHCS is a 16-block area in the neighborhood of the Columbia Presbyterian Medical Center, designated as Health Areas 3 and 4 of the Washington Heights Health District. Its population, according to the 1960 census, is composed of the following: Health Area 3, with a total population of 22,000, includes 1.6% Negroes, 5% Puerto Ricans, and 93.4% white; Health Area 4, with a total population of 26,000, includes 7.4% Negroes, 17% Puerto Rican, and 76% white. It is a residential area of multifamily dwellings and local businesses. The establishment of the WHCS was designed to provide facilities for psychiatric hospital care for all residents of this area. To ensure that patients would receive the appropriate available treatment, all admissions except readmissions were channeled through the Emergency Room and Outpatient Department of the Presbyterian Hospital or were transferred from Bellevue Hospital. It was hoped that utilization of the admission facilities of the Presbyterian Hospital would circumvent the transportation and admission of patients to Bellevue Hospital, some ten miles from the local area.

This new program led to a major reorganization of the clinical services of the Psychiatric Institute. The adult services, which were previously on one floor with a convalescent ward on another floor of the hospital, were changed to provide for the Washington Heights service and a general clinical service, each now having male and female patients. Furthermore, the services were physically relocated, each of the new services having all its component parts on a single floor of the hospital.

This arrangement allows for continuous nursing care from acute through convalescent care, and eliminates the numerous complications that occur when patients are moved from one floor to another, thereby distinctly categorizing them in terms of admission or convalescent status. On one floor of the WHCS, there is a mixing of all diagnostic and age groups, of brief-, medium-, and long-term patients, and of those who are day- or night-status patients.

A major goal of the new Service is to facilitate continuity of care by the same staff as well as by the same facility. To accomplish this the staff is divided into two therapeutic teams, each consisting of a supervising psychiatrist, residents, nurses, social workers, occupational therapists, and trainees of those paramedical groups. The newly admitted patient is assigned to a therapeutic team and remains with that team throughout all phases of treatment, including inpatient, day and night care, outpatient care, and subsequent readmission.

Each of the therapeutic teams is divided into two groups, which become the functioning therapeutic units and provide for an intimate relationship between staff and patients. Furthermore, whenever possible, staff offices are located on the floor, thus encouraging staff-patient contact as well as constantly introducing family members onto the floor during visits with the social workers and other staff.

Patients and therapeutic staff meet each morning to consider problems arising in the group. Relationships of patients with one another and with the staff are examined, privileges and passes granted, and interpersonal transactions with the group examined. Much emphasis is placed on involving the patient group in meaningful current activities designed to bring to the fore areas of healthy functioning as well as those affected by psychopathology.

The WHCS is self-contained, including an eight-bed intensive-care unit designed to provide for acutely disturbed patients. A Home Care Program is also provided in which family aides, who also serve as attendants, can assist patients in the hospital, during the transition to home, and at home. An attempt is made to provide home care services that will make the significant difference in improving adjustment within the community, thereby shortening and preventing hospitalization.

Working relationships exist with community agencies, including a consultation service for the local welfare department office. Obtaining welfare support for patients is facilitated by our participation in the application process. Because of the focus on clinical services to seriously ill patients, work with community agencies was concentrated on treatment programs for individual patients. In addition to the welfare department, these agencies include visiting nurse services to outpatients, vocational rehabilitation and training, sheltered workshops, and public schools. These ad hoc arrangements with regard to individual patients establish a pattern of collaboration that sets a foundation for the later development of broader programs, which can be expanded and focused on the less seriously ill in the community.

Method

Various procedures were established for the routine collection of data by each major staff member who is in contact with the patient and his family. The psychiatric resident, upon completion of his admission work-up, utilizes the Psychiatric Evaluation Form to make scaled judgments of various dimensions of psychopathology and characteristics of the patient's present illness. Demographic and other identifying information is obtained by the social worker and recorded on the Social Background Record. The psychiatric nurse makes ratings of 18 dimensions of psychopathology, using the Comprehensive Psychopathology Scales, the same scales used by the resident. Finally, research interviewers evaluate each new admission within the first few days of hospitalization, using the Psychiatric Status Schedule. This instrument consists of a structured interview schedule designed to obtain information from the patient regarding his feelings and behavior during the preceding week. Behavior during the interview also is noted, and all judgments are recorded in an inventory consisting of 492 items, which describe relatively small units of psychopathologic behavior.

The Psychiatric Evaluation Form, the Psychiatric Status Schedule, and the Comprehensive Psychopathology Scales all cover the following 17 dimensions, 13 of which rely heavily on previous factor analytic studies:[6] Inappropriate or Bizarre Appearance or Behavior; Belligerence-Negativism; Agitation-Excitement; Retardation-Emotional Withdrawal; Speech Disorganization; Suspicion-Persecution-Hallucinations; Grandiosity; Depression-Anxiety; Suicide-Self-Mutilation; Somatic Concerns; Social Isolation; Daily Routine–Leisure

Time Impairment; Sociopathic Impulses or Acts; Alcohol Abuse; Narcotic or Drug Abuse; Disorientation-Memory, and Denial of Illness.

The Psychiatric Status Schedule and the Psychiatric Evaluation Form also cover impairment in the roles of Wage Earner, House-keeper, Student, Mate, and Parent.

To ascertain whether the seriously mentally ill in this community were actually receiving the services offered, a case register was used to obtain information about admissions from this area to the principal alternative receiving facility, Bellevue Hospital. The case register provided data on the number of admissions to Bellevue Hospital from this catchment area, length of hospital stay, diagnosis, and disposition.

This study focused on a one-year period—September 1, 1965, to August 31, 1966. During this period there were 171 admissions to the WHCS, representing 152 different individuals. The data reported here is for the entire 171 admissions. Information from the Psychiatric Status Schedule was obtained on 130 admissions. The remaining patients were not interviewed because either they were too disturbed, no interviewer was available, or they had been interviewed during the previous two months, or the Spanish-speaking interviewer was not available.

Information from the Psychiatric Evaluation Form was obtained for the last 69 admissions after the Form was introduced in the middle of the year.

Results

The demographic characteristics of the 171 admissions are shown in Tables 1, 2, and 3.

Table 1 shows that one third of the admissions are in the adolescent and young adult group, ages 15 to 24. Over one half are below the age of 35. Five were in the over-65 group. There is a heavy preponderance of females to males, in the ratio of 2 to 1. Almost half the total have never been married, a figure compatible with the age distribution. Thirteen percent are nonwhite.

Table 2 shows the religious background, country of birth, and major ancestry. Over one half of the admissions are Catholic, one fourth Jewish, and the majority of the remainder Protestant. Almost half are foreign-born. One fifth were born in Puerto Rico. Examination of the breakdown by major ancestry shows the group to be heterogeneous, with a significant proportion coming from Puerto Rico, Ireland, and Europe.

TABLE 1

Selected Demographic Characteristics of WHCS Patients

Age	%	Marital Status	%
15–24	33	Single	45
25–34	25	Married	32
35–44	18	Widowed	8
45–54	11	Divorced	6
55–64	9	Separated	9
Over 65	5	RACE	
SEX	%	White	88
Male	33	Negro	12
Female	67	Other	1

TABLE 2

Selected Demographic Characteristics of WHCS Patients

Religious Background	%	Major Ancestry	%
Catholic	55	Continental U.S.	26
Protestant	16	Puerto Rico	22
Jewish	25	Ireland	12
Greek Orthodox	4	Germany	8
COUNTRY OF BIRTH		Russia	6
		Poland	2
Continental U.S.	58	Other Western European	13
Puerto Rico	19	Eastern Europe	2
Ireland	5	Mexico-Central-South America	4
Other Western European	5	Caribbean	5
Other	13		

The social class, type of admission, number of previous admissions, and the last stop before being admitted to the hospital are shown in Table 3. Eighty percent of the admissions were fairly evenly distributed in social classes III, IV, and V. Three quarters of the admissions were informal or voluntary, reflecting the emphasis on encouraging noncoercive admission procedures. For almost half the admissions, this was the first psychiatric hospitalization; 22%

TABLE 3

Selected Demographic Characteristics of WHCS Patients

Social Class (Hollingshead)	%	Previous Admissions	%
		None	44
I	4	One	20
II	8	Two	14
III	27	Three	7
IV	31	Four or More	15
V	22		
Uncoded	9		
TYPE OF ADMISSION	%	LAST STOP	%
Informal	26	P.H. Emergency Room	58
Voluntary	48	V.C. Psychiatric Clinic	4
1 P.C.	1	Bellevue	10
2 P.C.	9	Home	19
Return from C.C.	16	Other	9

had three or more. Most of the patients were admitted from the Emergency Room of the Presbyterian Hospital. Ten percent were transferred from Bellevue Hospital.

An examination of the interrelationships of the demographic information reveals an association between low social class, Puerto Rican ancestry, and Catholic religion. There is no association between number of previous admissions and social class. There is a tendency for women to have had more admissions than men.

Distribution by diagnoses made by the attending psychiatrist after the admission conference is shown in Table 4. Over half the admissions were diagnosed as schizophrenic reactions. Affective psychoses, neuroses, and personality disorders each accounted for approximately 10%. Only 4% were classified as acute or chronic brain syndrome.

The psychopathologic characteristics of this patient group can best be appreciated by comparing them with other groups expected to differ in both quantity and type of psychopathology. The mean standard scale scores* are presented in Figure 1. These groups are presented here merely for gross comparisons, recognizing that they

---

* The Standard scores used in this figure are based upon the mean and standard deviation of the pooled data from the four contrasting groups.

Fig. 1: Mean Standard Scores of Four Groups on the Factor Based Scales of the Psychiatric Status Schedule

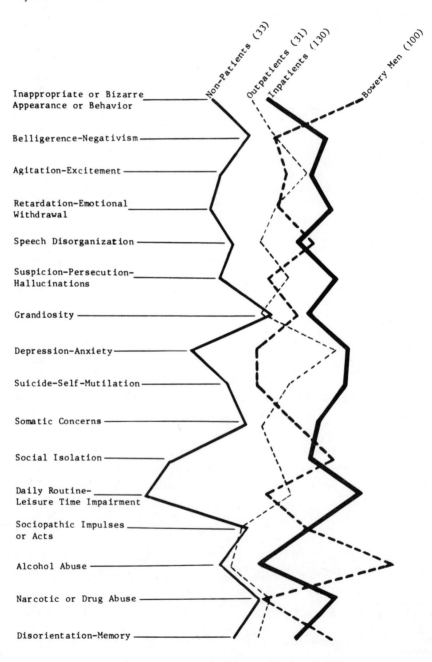

TABLE 4

Admission Conference Diagnosis

Diagnosis		%
Acute Brain Syndrome		1.75
Chronic Brain Syndrome		1.83
Affective Psychosis		8.18
Schizophrenic Reaction		56.14
Simple	2.92	
Hebephrenic	.58	
Catatonic	2.34	
Paranoid	19.30	
Acute Undifferentiated	5.85	
Chronic Undifferentiated	22.81	
Schizo-Affective	2.34	
Neuroses		12.86
Anxiety Reaction	3.51	
Conversion Reaction	.58	
Depression Reaction	8.77	
Personality Disorder		12.28
Inadequate Personality	.58	
Antisocial	2.34	
Alcoholism	2.34	
Drug Addiction	7.02	

are not matched on such variables as age, ethnicity, social class, etc.

The study group of 130 inpatients is represented by the heavy solid line. The thinner solid line depicts 33 non-patients living in the Washington Heights area. The broken line denotes 100 men interviewed at the Municipal Shelter in the Bowery section of New York. The dotted line labeled "Outpatients" represents 31 individuals seen approximately two years previously at a psychiatric outpatient clinic in the Washington Heights area.*

The WHCS group had higher scores than the outpatients and non-patients on all scales. As might be expected, the Bowery men scored significantly higher than the WHCS group on two scales: Inappropriate or Bizarre Appearance or Behavior, and Alcohol Abuse. The

* The data from the Psychiatric Status Schedule on the non-patients and outpatients has been provided by Bruce Dohrenwend, PhD. It represents only an initial portion of data being collected by him in his studies of the Washington Heights area of New York City. This represents early returns from a much larger sample and therefore is not a systematic sample. The interpretation of the data in the paper is made by the authors alone.

three scales that best discriminate between the WHCS group and the community non-patients are, in order of magnitude: Daily Routine–Leisure Time Impairment, Depression-Anxiety, and Social Isolation. (Epsilons of .43, .43, and .30 respectively.)

The scales that best discriminate between the WHCS group and the outpatients are Daily Routine–Leisure Time Impairment, Sociopathic Impulses or Acts, and Narcotic or Drug Abuse. (Epsilons of .15, .13, and .13.)

On one item of the Psychiatric Evaluation Form, the treating psychiatric resident is asked to indicate the one psychopathologic factor most instrumental in precipitating admission, using the same 17 dimensions as the Psychiatric Status Schedule Scales. The most common factors were Depression-Anxiety (20%); Suicide-Self-Mutilation (18%); Inappropriate or Bizarre Appearance or Behavior (12%); Alcohol Abuse, Belligerence-Negativism, and Agitation-Excitement were each noted for 9% of the patient group. Although the most differentiating scale on the Psychiatric Status Schedule was Daily Routine–Leisure Time Impairment, this dimension was noted as a precipitating factor for admission by the psychiatric resident for only 4% of the patients. This may be partially accounted for by a tendency on the part of the psychiatrist to subsume the impairment in daily routine under the symptomatology causing the impairment, principally depression.

The psychopathologic characteristics of the WHCS group can be further examined by inspecting the frequency of specific items in the Psychiatric Status Schedule inventory. Percentage notations are of the total patient group.

1. Depression-Anxiety. This area revealed the greatest frequency of items. Seventy persons admitted they were "often anxious," and 75% admitted they were "often sad or depressed." Seventy percent indicated they brooded "over certain unpleasant thoughts, feelings, or circumstances." Sixty-nine percent admitted they "felt like crying." Fifty-three percent indicated they "had trouble sleeping."

2. Suicide–Self-Mutilation. On this dimension, 32% indicated "thoughts about killing himself." A recent suicide attempt was noted in 15%. For 32% of the patients other people were judged to be "concerned that he might physically injure himself."

3. Social Isolation. In the area of Social Isolation, 39% indicated they "often avoid or fear contact or involvement with other people." Thirty percent indicated they "feel they have practically no friends or that they have little if any contact with friends."

4. Suspicion-Persecution-Hallucinations. In the dimension of Suspicion-Persecution-Hallucinations, 39% indicated they "cannot trust other people or are unduly suspicious of their intent." Nineteen percent had auditory hallucinations. Notably, an equal percent had olfactory hallucinations. Nine percent had visual hallucinations. Thirteen percent indicated persecutory delusions of being "attacked, harassed, cheated or persecuted." Fifteen percent indicated that "they take or plan to take action in response to some delusional belief."

5. Belligerence-Negativism. In the area of Belligerence-Negativism, 30% indicated they have "visible rages or fits of anger" (not including momentary verbal outbursts). For 18%, it was judged that other people "are concerned that he might physically injure another person."

6. Daily Routine–Leisure Time Impairment. In the area of Daily Routine–Leisure Time Impairment, 41% indicated that "his preoccupation, daydreaming, or bothersome thoughts interfere with the performance of his daily routine." Thirty-nine percent claimed they were "unable to perform at job, school, housework, or get anything done." Seventeen percent indicated that their "fears prevent them from participation in some activity." Twenty-two percent indicated they "often do not rise from sleep or nap when they intend."

7. Alcohol Abuse. Although only 4% were given an admission diagnosis of some form of alcoholism, 12% admitted "alcohol may be a problem for him." Nine percent admitted that "at times he keeps drinking even though he wants to stop or feels he should stop." Twelve percent admitted that "at times he skips an entire meal because he is drinking."

8. Narcotic or Drug Abuse. In the area of Drug Abuse, 14% indicated they "take one or more narcotics, narcotic-containing substances or consciousness-expanding drugs in the absence of a specific medical indication." Eight percent had been taking heroin, 10% marijuana, and 2% LSD or other hallucinogenic drugs.

Thirty-five percent of the total group—45 admissions—were judged to be potential wage-earners who were not working in the week prior to admission. Eighty-nine percent of these had the item: "Primarily because of his psychopathology, he has not worked at any time during the last week." Forty-two percent had "primarily because of his psychopathology, he has accepted his unemployment status, ie, he makes no serious effort to find work."

To what extent did the service meet the needs of those individuals who required psychiatric hospitalization during this one-year period? To answer this, the case registry was used to determine the number of hospitalizations from Health Areas 3 and 4 to both the WHCS and to Bellevue Hospital. Private hospitalization and direct admission to state hospitals are not included. It is our impression that the number of individuals involved in these groups is relatively small.

Admissions to the WHCS are divided into direct admissions and transfers from Bellevue Hospital.

TABLE 5

Hospital Admissions from Health Areas 3 and 4

9/1/65–8/31/66

	WHCS		BELLEVUE
	Direct	Bellevue Transfer	
Area	Number	Number	Number
3	62	4	30
4	64	13	70
Total	126	17	100

Total Hospitalizations = 226 (not including transfers)

During the first year there were 126 admissions from the community directly to the WHCS. There were also 100 admissions from the community to Bellevue Hospital, 17 of which were ultimately transferred to the WHCS. Thus, of the total hospitalizations from this community of 226, not including transfers, 83 (or 37%) went to Bellevue Hospital and were never served by the WHCS.

Of the patients admitted to Bellevue, 30 were discharged from that hospital, 24 were transferred to Rockland State Hospital, 17 were transferred to the WHCS, nine were prisoners, two went to non-state hospitals, 11 entered various other state hospitals, and three died. The disposition of four was unknown.

The annual number of hospitalizations from Health Areas 3 and 4 for three periods—Bellevue 1961, Bellevue 1964, and Bellevue and WHCS 1965/66—is shown in Table 6.

There was an increase in 1964 over 1961, but the combined WHCS and Bellevue hospitalizations for 1965 greatly exceed the Bellevue

TABLE 6

Annual Hospitalizations from Health Areas 3 and 4

	Bellevue 1961	Bellevue 1964	WHCS and Bellevue 1965
Area	Number	Number	Number
3	39	57	92
4	98	107	134
Total	137	164	226

1964 figure. Although it is difficult to determine the specific reasons for this larger increase, it is likely that it involves such factors as differences in admission policy of the Presbyterian Hospital admission service and greater utilization of the community-located facility.

To determine how the group actually served differed from the group seen at Bellevue, a comparison was made of the two groups on information that was available relative to both. Selected comparisons on which there were differences are shown in Table 7.

TABLE 7

Selected Comparison WHCS and Bellevue Admissions

	Bellevue %	WHCS %
Negro	19	12
Female	40	67
Over 65	14	5
Alcoholism	10	4
Senile or CAS	8	1.5

The Bellevue group had a higher incidence of Negroes, males, patients over 65, diagnoses of alcoholism, and senile or cerebro-arteriosclerotic brain syndrome (CAS).

There are several reasons why many individuals who went to Bellevue never were served by the WHCS. The ambulance service available to psychiatric patients in the Washington Heights community is directed to transport patients to Bellevue Hospital. The occasional unavailability of beds in the WHCS introduced a selective factor in transfers from Bellevue, thus tending to exclude those whose hospitalization might be brief, or those who would be transferred to a nursing home, or those who might require chronic care. Furthermore, the liaison with Bellevue was at times ineffective in reporting to the WHCS the admission of patients from its catchment area.

Discussion

The data presented indicates that the Washington Heights Community Service (WHCS) is dealing with a group of patients who are heterogeneous in social class, ancestry, chronicity, diagnosis, and areas of psychopathology. It shows an unusually heavy representation of women. Because of recent efforts to decrease the number of patients from this area admitted to Bellevue Hospital, it is anticipated that the WHCS group will increase in number and in acuteness of illness. There will be more patients with problems associated with alcoholism and with aging. The sex ratio undoubtedly will shift toward the usual distribution of females having only a slight preponderance over males.

This data has implications for planning and organization of services. The method of organization of treatment modalities is supported in part by the data indicating the major areas of psychopathology of the patient population.

Daily Routine–Leisure Time Impairment and Social Isolation are treated by means of a variety of group activities. For example, the daily living groups emphasize difficulties our patients have in organizing and carrying out routine tasks of group living. They also focus on the utilization of hospital and community resources for leisure-time activities. Although some emphasis is placed on practical problems, major attention is given to the intrapsychic conflicts that interfere with effective utilization of available opportunities. Feelings of worthlessness, of social unacceptability, fears of rejection, inhibitions in assertiveness, and excessive dependency are revealed in the group process. Patients have a daily opportunity to observe these difficulties and to experiment with new and more effective means of adaptation. To increase the sense of competence and integration in the community, patients are encouraged to join such ward activities as consumer education groups, planned parenthood discussions, homemaking and child care groups, and community programs that include adult education courses and basic education skills such as reading, writing, and speaking the English language.

Depression-Anxiety, as well as other symptomatic expressions of psychopathology, are treated with drugs and individual psycho-therapy. Virtually all patients receive either one of the phenothia-zines or antidepressant medications at some time during their hospital stay. In addition, most patients remain on medication when they are followed as outpatients.

The psychotherapeutic focus utilizes the intimate and intensive daily contact of patients and staff, which provides the opportunity to observe each patient constantly and to evaluate his capacity for functioning, his areas of regression, and maladaptive behavior patterns. This focus on the "here and now" serves to intensify the meaningfulness of the treatment situations to both patient and staff as well as to elucidate those behavior patterns, both characterologic and symptomatic, which principally interfere with functioning. These observations provide a common ground for a discussion between therapist and patient. In this context, the historic derivation and factors influencing maladaptive behavior are made more meaningful to both patient and therapist. Such an approach is in accordance with reports made of the data-gathering and therapeutic value of observing family interactions and group process. This method of gathering and using observational data with regard to patient functioning makes possible effective psychotherapy with patients from all classes who have varying capacities verbally to report events, feelings, behavior, and symptoms. In such a setting, the usual procedure of regular psychotherapeutic sessions is, by and large, accepted and valued by the patient.[7]

Our experience with the heterogeneous population at the WHCS has indicated that not all patients can be effectively treated in a completely "open door" facility. An intensive care unit provides supervision and structure for the more acutely disturbed patient. This unit, however, is part of the ward, and patients in this unit participate in the regular group and ward activities as fully as their condition permits. This prevents the isolation of the acutely disturbed and the establishment of a separate culture for them.

The large number of patients who either have not been working or have serious problems relative to their work require special help. Additionally, in making vocational and career choices, many individuals in the socially disadvantaged groups have lacked the opportunity fully and effectively to utilize their intelligence and capacity. The opportunity for vocational training offered by the WHCS further suggests to the patient a staff attitude that he is capable of functioning at a higher level, which of course has a salutary effect.

The social complications involved in the illness of our patient group make heavy demands on the social service department. The degree of family disruption, problems in housing, welfare support, need for medical services, as well as for vocational training, require extensive social services. This demand is further increased as the families of patients view the hospital as an available facility for supplying a variety of needs. The families as well as the individual patients thus increase the work load of the Service.

The WHCS organization providing continuity of facilities—ie, inpatient, day and night, and outpatient care—and continuity of therapeutic staff, has numerous advantages. Patients can readily be moved from one status to another, depending on their clinical condition, with minimal administrative problems. The patient's relationships with staff members and other patients are not altered as his condition changes. Each patient has a constant view of the other patients, extending from those on intensive care to those working or attending school in the community. This we feel enhances the mobility of patients through the range of services.

Among the research possibilities in this community mental health service is the opportunity to study (1) the difference between patients and non-patients living in the same community; (2) the incidence of serious mental illness in a defined urban area; (3) the various problems associated with treating patients from the lower social classes; (4) the differential aspect of specific treatment modalities, such as comparing day versus full inpatient care, treatment by paramedical personnel, and individual, group, and drug treatments.

II THE SECOND YEAR'S EXPERIENCE

Program planning and evaluation require a continuous monitoring and study of the demographic and psychopathologic characteristics of the patient population combined with a study of the effects of administrative decisions. It can be stated that our impressions often have not been confirmed by the data. The amassing of data permits informed decision-making, flexibility in the treatment programs, and responsiveness to the needs of the community. As a result of the information collected during the first year of operation of the WHCS, various administrative changes were made to further the program's original goals.

Efforts were made to avoid hospitalization of catchment area patients at Bellevue Hospital. Patients arriving at Bellevue from our area were to be transferred immediately by ambulance to the WHCS on a seven-day-a-week, 24-hour basis. Although this plan appeared simple, numerous administrative and staffing problems with regard to ambulance services made it practically unworkable. Not one patient was transferred by ambulance from Bellevue to our Service. However, efforts with neighboring hospitals, Presbyterian Hospital, the police, and—most important—our own psychiatric residents were more successful. The number of admissions to Bellevue from the catchment area decreased from 100 during the first year to 67 during the second year. In the first year only 17% of those admitted to Bellevue were transferred to WHCS, but in the second year 45% were so transferred. Many of the remainder were discharged from Bellevue directly back to the community.

Our established initial policy was to admit patients whenever possible under an informal admission status. However, the first year showed only 26% of the admissions being of this type. We discovered that the admitting resident and the nursing supervisor preferred the voluntary status because it gave the staff greater control. The informal-admission-status rate rose to 58% when the admitting staff's anxiety was overcome.

Assuming responsibility for a particular catchment area makes it necessary to establish a policy of excluding out-of-area patients. During the first year 25% of the admissions were from outside the catchment area; during the second year the figure dropped to 11%. This small percentage were considered elective admissions for teaching purposes and worthwhile exceptions to the general admission policy.

A decision was made in the second year routinely to collect information on patient movement through various statuses—day, night, and OPD—the length of stay in these statuses, the treatments received, and the disposition when they left. This information was recorded on our Change of Status Record.

During a 12-month period (7/66 through 6/67), the mean length of stay for inpatients was approximately 12 weeks. The median was only 5.5 weeks, however, because of the large number of patients leaving within the first (modal) week. A trend toward shorter admissions became apparent when, during the first six months, approximately 28% left inpatient status during the first week, whereas during the last six months the figure was 36%.

Treatments were categorized as milieu, group psychotherapy, individual psychotherapy, family, and somatic therapy. Of the 176 patients who left inpatient status, 78% were treated with drugs. This mode of treatment was judged to be the major treatment for 35%. Individual psychotherapy was given to 82% of the patients, but was considered the major treatment modality for only 32%. Though virtually all patients were involved in the milieu program, it was considered the major treatment program for 24%. Group psychotherapy and family treatment were received by 55% and 21% respectively, but rarely were considered a major treatment modality. These data indicate that with this varied patient population, plus the current orientation of our residents and attending staff, an approximately equal number of patients are judged to have had as the major treatment modality either milieu, individual psychotherapy, or drugs.

A few changes became necessary in our data collection procedures. The nurses had difficulty making the scaled judgments of the Comprehensive Psychopathology Scales; thus this procedure was eliminated. Most of the nurse difficulty, in this instance, appeared to be relative to lack of motivation, because of the pressure of other duties.

An examination of data from the Social Background Record, the Psychiatric Status Schedule, and the Psychiatric Evaluation Form revealed remarkable consistency in demographic and psychopathologic characteristics. Consistency also occurred in the distribution of diagnoses and in the number of previous admissions to the Psychiatric Institute or other facilities. Some notable exceptions to these consistencies, not previously mentioned, include a shift of the sex ratio from the previous 67% females during the first year to 52% during the second year, which was probably due to the increased admission of disturbed males who previously went to Bellevue and were not transferred. Although the age distribution did not change, there were a greater number of students admitted. Also, compared with the students admitted during the first year, these were significantly more impaired in their functioning as students ($P<.01$). Finally, suicide or self-mutilation as the primary reason for admission increased from 18% to 27%, this being reflected in higher scores in this dimension on the Psychiatric Status Schedule ($P<.05$).

SUMMARY

This two-year study has described the demographic characteristics of a patient population from a specific catchment area, their psychopathologic characteristics, the degree to which a community service has fulfilled its declared policy of providing psychiatric hospitalization for all those who require it, and efforts to develop treatment programs responsive to the needs of the patient group. A major next step is the evaluation of the various components of the treatment armamentarium. There is a salutary "catch" in the concept of catchment area. The catchment area concept, which emphasizes treatment of the patient in his local area, provides an opportunity and an obligation for such evaluation. The coupling of responsibility for care and evaluation will permit careful scrutiny of the promise for and the results of community mental health services.

REFERENCES

1. Lendt, L. A.: Social History of Washington Heights, New York City. Mimeographed working paper with limited distribution, February 1960.
2. Bemmels, V. G.: Survey of Mental Health Problems in Social Caseloads, *Amer. J. Psych.*, 121:136–147 (No. 2), August 1964.
3. Fisch, M., Gruenberg, E. M., and Bandfield, C.: Epidemiology of Psychiatric Emergencies in an Urban Health District, *Amer. J. Public Health*, 54:572–579 (No. 4), April 1964.
4. Mesnikoff, A. M., and Peretz, D.: Evolution of Community-Based Mental Health Orientation on University Psychiatric Service, read before the Divisional Meeting of American Psychiatric Association, New York City, November 9, 1963.
5. Dohrenwend, B. P.: Some Aspects of Appraisal of Abnormal Behavior by Leaders in Urban Area, *Amer. Psychol.*, 17:190–198 (No. 4), 1962.
6. Spitzer, R. L., et al: Mental Status Schedule: Properties of Factor Analytically Derived Scales, *Arch. Gen. Psychiat.*, 16:479–493, 1967.
7. Mesnikoff, A. M.: Therapeutic Milieu for the Seriously Disturbed, *Int. Psychiat. Clin.*, 1 (No. 4), October 1964.

5

The Walk-In Service:
An Experience in Community Care*

by RICHARD I. SHADER

Dr. Shader carefully analyzes the aims, disposition of treatment, care of patients in terms of social class, and the other variables of the Walk-In-Service. He shows that the population and the disposition of the patients depend more frequently on the built-in biases of the mental health administration and workers rather than on the needs of the patient.

P. Janet was the first to note that if a patient is disturbed and is poor, he is sent to a mental hospital and is called psychotic; if he is middle class, he goes to a sanatorium with nurses and doctors because he is psychasthenic; if a patient is rich, he stays at home with family and servants, has a private physician, and is called eccentric.

Shader's results confirm Janet's concept, revealing how the clinicians' bias shapes therapeutic strategy. Both social class and diagnosis were related to the type of treatment initially assigned and actually received. Higher social class applicants and neurotic applicants were more frequently offered some form of treatment at the Massachusetts Mental Health Center. Other patients were sent to centers considered less prestigious.

More studies of this type are needed to describe the behavior of investigators and clinicians.

Public health approaches have become central concerns for contemporary American psychiatry. Attesting to this fact are the pro-

* Presented at the Annual Meeting of the American College of Neuropsychopharmacology, Puerto Rico, December 1966.

Supported in part by grants from the Harrington Fund, Harvard University; the Medical Foundation, Inc., Boston; USPHS Grant FR 0 5555-04.

grams in social and preventive psychiatry being developed in most training centers. The federal government and many states have enacted legislation to implement the construction and staffing of community mental health centers, the aim of such centers being to place diagnostic and treatment services within easy reach of the average citizen.

Among the many innovations introduced to provide more immediate and more comprehensive care have been day hospitals, home treatment services, suicide prevention centers, and psychiatric emergency services. One type of psychiatric emergency service is the walk-in clinic. Tannenbaum[1] has recently described the walk-in services of the Jacobi Hospital (Bronx Municipal Hospital of the City of New York and the Albert Einstein Medical Center) and of the Metropolitan Hospital (Department of Psychiatry of New York Medical College), whose clinics emphasize the value of brief psychotherapy and the importance of abolishing waiting lists.

Paralleling the developments at these institutions, an experimental emergency service was initiated at the Massachusetts Mental Health Center in 1960.[2] In 1961 the Emergency Service was made a formal component of the comprehensive facilities of this Center. It functioned for three years with approximately 700 new patients annually presenting varied problems: marital and job problems, panic states, suicidal feelings, traumatic sexual experiences, legal involvements, etc. In 1963, because of the successful functioning of the Emergency Service, it was decided that all applicants for outpatient care as well as emergencies would initially be seen according to a uniform "walk-in" intake procedure. Since that time an increasing number of applicants have been evaluated. In 1966 it was further decided that even applicants or referrals for inpatient care at the parent institution would first be evaluated at the Walk-In Service; 3,309 new cases were seen in 1967. These cases were in many ways similar to those seen from 1961 through 1963. However, the range has broadened and there are now more cases because of problems with aging, drug abuse (particularly LSD), or concerns about being eligible for the draft.

DESCRIPTION OF THE WALK-IN SERVICE

The Walk-In Service of the Southard Clinic, the outpatient facility of the Massachusetts Mental Health Center, shares with the parent institution the advantages of an unrestricted range of treatment modalities, exceptional staffing in terms of both the ratio of treating professionals to patients and of teaching supervisors to residents, unusually flexible arrangements for continuity of patient care, and a unified record system, which is especially simple in the case of the Clinic.[3] The structure of the Walk-In Service minimizes the influences of administrative procedure and traditions upon the initial encounter and subsequent contacts between the therapist and patient. Each individual applying for treatment at the Clinic (hereafter referred to as the "applicant") usually is given an initial consultation by a second-year psychiatric resident (hereafter referred to as the "interviewer"), who is assigned to walk-in shifts in rotation from about 25 residents available for this purpose. In addition, some cases are seen by social workers who are receiving advanced supervised training in the Clinic, by third-year residents who are receiving additional walk-in experience, and by medical students as part of their supervised clinical work.

The initial interview is uncontaminated by screening interviews, advance categorizations, preselections, or waiting lists. Thus, each applicant begins the initial interview with the interviewer afresh. Because applicants are seen immediately after arriving at the Clinic, the timing of the initial consultation is invariably determined by the applicant's felt need. Although only one quarter of our applicant population initially are in "crisis" in the sense of considering themselves emergency cases, all receive "crisis consultations" since they are seen when the need for help impels them to act. The interviewer tries to focus upon the issue that caused them to seek help.

The basic administrative and teaching philosophy of the Clinic is concerned with maximizing the role of the initially responsible professional person (the interviewer). Clinic policy is directed toward minimizing extra-clinical considerations as to dispositions. Thus, disposition for each case evolves mainly from within the relationship established in the initial consultation.

When the applicant first arrives at the Walk-In Service he presents himself to a receptionist, who obtains background information to start the clinical record. The applicant, who has been advised of procedure, then waits until one of the interviewers becomes available. Typically, an applicant is seen within 20 minutes. The length of the interview is determined by that day's Service work load and the time that the interviewer judges to be necessary to arrive at an understanding of the case. Senior staff supervisors are available to discuss cases with the interviewers. On occasion, an interviewer may request a supervisor to see the patient to help clarify any uncertainties about the case. The interviewer concludes the meeting with the applicant by working out future plans (disposition) with him. At the termination of the initial interview, the interviewer completes the clinical record by writing down his impressions of the case, historic material, and his diagnosis and disposition. A wide range of initial dispositions is available.

The procedure is graphically illustrated in Figure 1.

Most of these initial dispositions are self-explanatory. Several, however, require further clarification:

Extended Diagnostic Evaluation

The interviewer might feel that further sessions are required in order to arrive at a diagnosis or to work out a treatment plan. He might wish to evaluate the effects of the initial consultation before making decisions regarding further treatment. Extended diagnostic evaluations in practice usually last two to three visits, although they may be longer. This initial disposition is used for between 20% and 30% of the applicants.

Teaching Diagnostic Evaluation

Senior staff members conduct teaching sessions in which diagnostic techniques are taught to small groups of medical students or residents. Applicants with interesting diagnostic problems can be referred from the Walk-In Service for further evaluation. This disposition is used for between 5% and 20% of the applicants. Most teaching diagnostics are begun within three weeks following the initial walk-in visit.

Intermittent Supportive Therapy

About 2% of the applicants are referred directly from the Walk-In Service for long-term supportive therapy, usually on a once-a-month basis. Frequently such patients are on maintenance drug regimens. Some patients are referred for intermittent support following extended diagnostic study or after a teaching diagnostic evaluation. This increases the number of Walk-In Service applicants who receive intermittent supportive therapy to about 5% to 7%.

No Further Attention

After the initial walk-in visit, from 15% to 20% of walk-in patients are given a disposition of "no further attention." In such instances most applicants are advised to contact the interviewer again in the

Fig. 1: Pathways to Walk-In Consultation

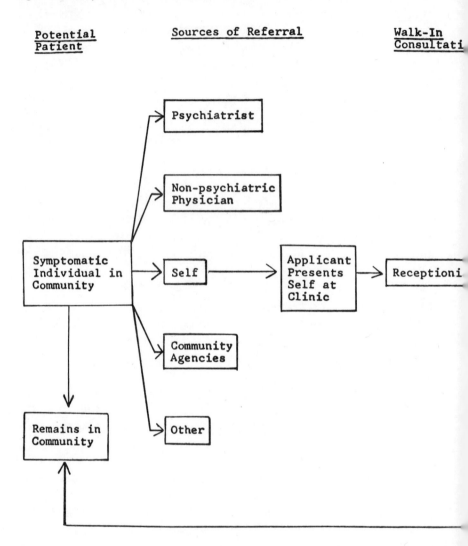

future should they feel the need for further help. A survey on 200 consecutive walk-in cases six months after the initial visit revealed that approximately 50% were receiving no further attention. This includes applicants who were terminated after extended diagnostic study, teaching diagnostic evaluations, or after the conclusion of short-term therapy.

Initial Disposition

Interview (Resident, Medical Student, Social Worker)

Intermittent Supportive Therapy

Group Therapy

Couples or Family Therapy

Short-term Therapy

Long-term Therapy

Teaching Diagnostic Evaluation

Extended Diagnostic Evaluation

MMHC Day Hospital

MMHC Full-time Hospital

Hospitalization Elsewhere

Return to Referring Individual or Agency

Private Psychiatric or Social Worker Referral

No Further Attention

Long-Term Therapy

About 4% of the applicants are referred for long-term individual psychotherapy directly following the initial walk-in visit. This percentage increases to about 15% six months following the initial visit. Included are cases referred after extended or teaching diagnostics, as well as a few cases who enter long-term treatment at the conclusion of short-term therapy. Patients in long-term therapy usually are seen once or twice a week for one to two years.

Short-Term Therapy

This goal-directed treatment is generally time-limited to eight to 12 visits. About 10% of the applicants are directly referred for short-term work. In a study of 500 consecutive cases, 9% were still in short-term therapy six months after their first visit. Some patients had completed their treatment by this time, but additional cases were begun at the conclusion of extended or teaching diagnostics. Of these 500 applicants, 48 applicants were initially referred for short-term therapy. Six months later, 15 were still in the process of completing their short-term therapy, eight had renegotiated goals and were now in long-term individual therapy, two had started group psychotherapy, one had been referred to a psychiatrist in private practice, three were receiving intermittent support, one was admitted to the Day Hospital at the Center, one was hospitalized on an inpatient service at the Center, four had been referred to community agencies, one was hospitalized at another local hospital, and 12 had completed their short-term therapy and were functioning adequately in the community.

Hospitalization

About 2% to 5% of walk-in applicants are referred directly to the Day Hospital at the Center; another 3% to 10% are hospitalized on one of three inpatient services at the Center, and 3% to 9% are referred for hospitalization elsewhere.

Use of Medications

About 10% of the applicants are given medications while under the care of the Walk-In Service.

RESEARCH IN THE WALK-IN SERVICE

In 1965 a number of studies were initiated in the Walk-In Service by the author in collaboration with William A. Binstock, MD. It was the goal of these studies to provide basic information about the functioning of the Walk-In Service and to learn more about the population being served. Three of these studies are summarized below.

The first study[4] was undertaken in order to understand the drug-prescribing behavior of the physicians in the Walk-In Service. For this study we focused on 100 consecutive cases diagnosed as non-psychotic depressive reactions, to determine what variables influenced residents' decisions to prescribe antidepressant medication. Of these 100 cases, 23 were given antidepressant medication (imipramine [Tofrānil] or amitriptypline [Elavil]). Before undertaking this study we made five predictions: (1) social class would be a relevant factor in drug use, with drugs more often being prescribed for the lower classes; (2) interviewer attitudes at the time of the initial consultation relative to drug decision would be based on liking for, less anger toward, and more optimism for patients as associated with less frequent use of drugs; (3) even with controls for social class, interviewer attitudes would still be linked to the drug decision; (4) more specifically, within a given class level drugs would not be used for the "more liked" patients; (5) gross estimates of manifest psychopathology at the time of the initial consultation would not differentiate between the drug and non-drug groups.

Each physician completed an attitude questionnaire at the conclusion of the initial walk-in interview. This questionnaire was used to assess the interviewer's conscious responses, such as his degree of optimism, liking, or anger toward the applicant. Each applicant completed the Langner 22-Item Symptom Scale. Neither residents nor applicants were aware of the hypotheses being tested.

Attitude Scale

The attitude scale[5, 6] contains 15 items. Each item is rated on a five-point scale (from 0 = "not at all" to 4 = "extremely"). For this study, we chose three items: (1) "How likable is this patient?" (2) "How angry are you at this patient?" (3) "How optimistic are you about this patient?" In addition, a six-item cluster score, derived by a factor analysis of the 15-item scale, was examined. This score was derived by adding scores from items 1 and 3 to the question "How much do you like being with this patient?" and then subtracting item 2, as well as the scores, from the questions: "How hopeless do you feel about the patient?" and "How much does this patient make you feel helpless or in a bind?" The six-item totals obtained ranged between -12 and $+12$, reflecting a positive-hopeful versus negative-subjective orientation toward the applicant.

Langner Scale

The Langner scale[7] is a 22-item self-rating scale of psychiatric symptoms indicating impairment. These items, which cover anxiety, somatic concerns, and depression, have been found to be effective in discriminating populations with varying degrees of psychiatric morbidity.

Social Class

Social class was determined from the demographic information by employing the Hollingshead-Redlich Two Factor Index of Social Position.[8]

Age, sex, and prescription of antidepressant medication were obtained from the record. The American Psychiatric Association diagnostic classification scheme is followed in the Walk-In Service.

Results

All social classes were represented in the study sample. However, to investigate the relationship between social class and drug use, classes 1 and 2 were pooled, as were classes 4 and 5. Drugs were prescribed for one of 19 patients in classes 1 and 2, one of 19 class 3 patients, and for 21 of 62 patients in classes 4 and 5. Chi-square analysis revealed that antidepressant medications were used significantly more often in lower-class patients ($P<.01$).

Chi-square analysis applied to data relative to drug use and interviewer attitudes supported our second prediction: Drug use was significantly associated with less liking for the patient ($P<.05$), and with increased anger toward the patient ($P<.05$). Optimism tended to be associated negatively with drug use, but did not reach statistical significance. The six-item composite score was negatively related to drug use, but indicated borderline statistical significance.

Our prediction that once having controlled for social class, we would find drug use a function of interviewer attitudes, could be tested only within classes 4 and 5. Chi-square analysis revealed that liking was significantly associated with drugs not being used in class 5 ($P<.01$). The results tended to be in the same direction in class 4, but did not reach statistical significance. Similarly, with the six-item composite score, negative attitudes were significantly linked to more frequent drug use in class 5 ($P<.05$), but not in class 4. None of the other comparisons reached statistical significance, though they were in the expected directions. Thus, although our findings were in the predicted direction, they were not sufficiently strong to support prediction 3. Our more specific prediction that the "more liked" patients would be given less drugs was clearly supported within class 5, but not within class 4.

Total Langner scores were examined for their relationship to drug use. There was no significant difference in level of impairment between the drug and no-drug groups, which is in support of prediction 5.

Comment

The results of this study indicated clear linkages between treatment assignments and the educational-economic background of the patients in our sample. A similar role can be ascribed to the doctor's subjective attitudes toward the patient. Our data also suggest that social class and doctor's attitudes toward the patient, although not synonymous, tend to co-vary in their contribution to the clinician's decisions. Since these factors are not part of the physician's conscious deliberations, we designate them as unconscious biases, even though lower-class patients often expect and prefer a nonpsychologic, medical approach.[9, 10]

In a second project, the 500 consecutive applicants previously mentioned were studied to investigate factors leading to the allocation of the wide range of dispositions available at the Walk-In Service.[11] Studies of psychiatric facilities frequently indicate that the social class of the potential patient is a powerful determinant of the amount and type of help he receives, despite the fact that those planning, administering, and working in these facilities do not intend social class per se to play such an important role.[12-19]

A number of studies[19-24] of traditional outpatient treatment settings have evaluated the relationships among social characteristics of patients, therapists' assessments of patients' motivation for therapy, and the relationships between such assessments and the therapists' attitudes toward patients. It has been suggested, however, that "the frequent non-correspondence of results among such studies attests to the need for further research clarifying the relation of various personal variables to the selection of clinic patients and to the length and outcome of their therapeutic treatment."[14]

Other studies of outpatient settings suggest that factors such as stimulating a positive reaction in the screening physician or therapist, the therapist's liking for the patient, and the presence of warmth in the therapeutic interaction are related to both the selection of patients for treatment and the outcome of treatment.[22-24]

These findings support the significance of social class, liking, and optimism as relevant parameters in any study of the determinants of disposition. Yet selection for treatment is traditionally expected to be determined by diagnosis.

Almost all these studies focused mainly on selection for long-term individual psychotherapy. It was our hypothesis that attitudes and social class would be associated with disposition to the extent that forms of treatment involving more dyadic interactions would be assigned to upper social class and more liked applicants. Similarly, we expected that the more liked applicants and upper social class applicants would more frequently be offered some form of treatment at the parent institution, whereas lower-class or less liked applicants would be referred elsewhere or given no further attention. Further, we predicted that lower-class or less liked applicants would be more frequently hospitalized. Diagnosis was also examined as a function of attitudes and social class and as a determinant of disposition. Thus, the four major variables being considered were (1) Social Class of the Applicant; (2) Attitude of the Interviewer Toward the Applicant; (3) Diagnosis; and (4) Disposition.

For this study, we used only the six-item attitude cluster described in our first study.[4] The dispositions included the categories listed in Figure 1. Disposition was evaluated twice: the plan at the conclusion of the initial interview; and what actually happened to the applicant within the first six months following the initial interview.

Results

Chi-square analyses were used to assess the relationships among the major variables. The results largely confirmed the hypotheses being tested. A significant trend emerged, which can be summarized as follows: Both diagnosis and social class were related to the type of treatment initially assigned and actually received, whereas interviewer attitude determined whether the treatment would be at the Center or elsewhere. For example, lower social class applicants and non-neurotic applicants were more frequently hospitalized. More liked applicants were more frequently. offered some form of treatment at the Center.

A third study[25] focused on the applicants who failed to return when extended diagnostic study had been suggested. In brief, lower social class applicants were more frequently found in this non-return group, and the non-return group had more frequently elicited some degree of anger in the interviewer.

DISCUSSION

The Walk-In Service is now well established as the interface between the community and the Massachusetts Mental Health Center. Although other walk-in clinics emphasize short-term individual psychotherapy, the unusually large staffing arrangements at the Center make available a wide range of possible treatments. Hence, thorough and immediate evaluation is the emphasis of the Walk-In Service at the Center. From the research conducted it would appear that the influence of social class per se has been minimized, since it does not determine whether the applicant is eventually treated at the Center. However, initial interviewer attitudes may determine whether or not the applicant will be offered treatment at the Center.

It has also become clear that, paralleling the expansion and refinement of the services of the Walk-In Service, there has been an increase in requests for service from the community. Increasing efforts currently are being directed toward the development of consultative services or liaison with a variety of community organizations and agencies.

The Walk-In Service also provides an excellent opportunity for training. Residents, medical students, social workers, psychologists, and other care-giving professionals have the opportunity to treat or observe a wide variety of problems. One of the first issues to be faced, however, concerns which applicants should become patients. This issue has recently been discussed by Levinson, Merrifield, and Berg.[26] In other words, to whom do we offer more than the initial evaluation? Who is best served by remaining a non-patient?

Another interesting problem posed in this setting is the evaluation of suicidal risk or potential. Many applicants present themselves fairly soon following an emotional crisis. Although this may maximize therapeutic leverage, it also increases the number of applicants who are in the high-risk, three-month period following such crises.[27] In all walk-in evaluations it is essential to learn: Why has the applicant come in at this particular time? Who are the important objects in his life, and what is the current nature of their relationships? What alternatives does he feel are open to him, and how does *he* feel he can best be helped?

Walk-in clinics have definitely come of age in the 1960s. Additional refinements and elaborations are essential and inevitable. One of the challenges to be met will be adequate staffing, and further work must be done to find alternatives to traditional staffing patterns. Let us hope such solutions and facilities will be more widely available by the 1970s.

REFERENCES

1. Tannenbaum, G.: "Walk-In Clinic," in Arieti, S. (ed.): *American Handbook of Psychiatry*, New York: Basic Books, 1966, vol. 3, pp. 577–587.
2. Greenblatt, M.: "Mental Hospital as Community Extension Service," in Greenblatt, M., et al: *Prevention of Hospitalization*, New York: Grune & Stratton, 1963.
3. Glasscote, R. M., et al: *Community Mental Health Center—Analysis of Existing Models*, Washington, D.C.: Joint Information Service, 1964.
4. Shader, R. I., Binstock, W. A., and Scott, D.: Suggestive Determinants of Drug Prescription: Study of Therapists' Attitudes, *Hosp. Community Psychiat.*, 19:34–37 (12), 1968.
5. Kellam, S. G., Durell, J., and Shader, R. I.: Nursing Staff Attitudes and the Clinical Course of Psychotic Patients, *Arch. Gen. Psychiat.*, 14:190–202, 1966.
6. Shader, R. I., Kellam, S. G., and Durell, J.: Social Field Events During First Week of Hospitalization as Predictors of Treatment Outcome for Psychotic Patients, *J. Nerv. Ment. Dis.*, 145:142–153, 1967.
7. Langner, T.: Twenty-two Item Screening Score of Psychiatric Symptoms Indicating Impairment, *J. Health Human Behav.*, 3:269–276, Winter 1962.
8. Hollingshead, A. B., and Redlich, F. C.: *Social Class and Mental Illness*, New York: John Wiley & Sons, 1958.
9. Yamamoto, J., and Goin, M.D.: Social Class Factors Relevant for Psychiatric Treatment, *J. Nerv. Ment. Dis.*, 142:332–339 (4), April 1966.
10. Aronson, H., and Overall, B.: Treatment Expectations of Patients in Two Social Classes, *Social Work*, 11:35–41, January 1966.
11. Shader, R. I., Binstock, W. A., Ohly, J. I., and Scott, D.: Biasing Factors in Diagnosis and Disposition, *Comp. Psychiat.*, 10 (No. 2), 81–89, 1969.
12. Albronda, H. D., Dean, R. L., and Starkweather, V. A.: Social Class and Psychotherapy, *Arch. Gen. Psychiat.*, 10:276–283, 1964.
13. Auld, F., Jr., and Myers, J. K.: Contributions to Theory for Selecting Psychotherapy Patients, *J. Clin. Psychol.*, 10:56–60, 1954.
14. Brown, J. S., and Kosterlitz, N.: Selection and Treatment of Psychiatric Outpatients, *Arch. Gen. Psychiat.*, 11:425–437, 1964.
15. Cole, N., Branch, C. H., and Allison, R. B.: Some Relationships Between Social Class and Practice of Dynamic Psychotherapy, *Amer. J. Psychiat.*, 118:1004–1012, 1962.
16. Hollingshead, A. B., and Redlich, F. C.: *Social Class and Mental Illness*, New York: John Wiley & Sons, 1958.
17. Levinson, D. J., Gallagher, E. B.: *Patienthood in Mental Hospital*, Boston: Houghton Mifflin, 1964.
18. Schaffer, L., and Myers, J. K.: Psychotherapy and Social Stratification, *Psychiatry*, 17:83–93, 1954.
19. Shyne, A. W.: What Research Tells Us about Short-Term Cases in Family Agencies, *Social Casework*, May 1957.
20. Rosenthal, D., and Frank, J. D.: Fate of Psychiatric Clinic Outpatients Assigned to Psychotherapy, *J. Nerv. Ment. Dis.*, 127:330–343, 1958.
21. Jones, O., and Speck, R. V.: Psychotherapy in Adult Outpatient Clinic, *Penn. Psychiat. Quart.*, 27–38, 1961.
22. Brill, N. W., and Storrow, H. A.: Social Class and Psychiatric Treatment, *Arch. Gen. Psychiat.*, 3:340–344, 1960.
23. Strupp, J. M., et al: Psychotherapists' Assessment of Former Patients, *J. Nerv. Ment. Dis.*, 137:220–230, 1963.

24. Wallach, M.: Judgments of Motivations for Psychotherapy: Some Further Explorations. Unpublished data, 1964.
25. Salzman, C., Shader, R. I., and Scott, D.: Unpublished data, 1967.
26. Levinson, D. J., Merrifield, J., and Berg, K.: Becoming a Patient, *Arch. Gen. Psychiat.*, 17:385–406, 1967.
27. Schneidman, E. S., and Farberow, N. L.: Suicide—The Problem and Its Magnitude, *Med. Bull. Veterans Admin.*, MB-7, March 1961.

PERSPECTIVES
IN THE TREATMENT
OF SCHIZOPHRENIA

6

Hospitalization of Schizophrenic Patients: Prediction and Prevention*

by DAVID M. ENGELHARDT
and REUBEN A. MARGOLIS

For a number of years Engelhardt and Margolis performed an investigation of the phenothiazine prevention of hospitalization of the schizophrenic patient, and discovered a relatively small number were prone to hospitalization. A further study was made of the variables associated with community care and rehospitalization. A scale was devised to predict the hospitalization-proneness (HPS). Variables were scored so that a high HPS score represented the non-prone, whereas a low score represented the patient prone to hospitalization. The findings that resulted were statistically significant, including evidence that phenothiazines, especially chlorpromazine, are effective in altering both time and rate of hospitalization in the chronic schizophrenic outpatient. The HPS has proved a valuable research tool. By identifying the prone and non-prone patient, Engelhardt and Margolis were able to establish differential drug effects for these two populations; also, to identify positive and negative drug effects.

This study is highly significant to the understanding of the following chapter by Rothman. His special subtype of early, acute schizophrenic patient was rarely rehospitalized, and the patient's own choice of treat-

* The authors wish to acknowledge the contribution of Drs. Norbert Freedman, Leon D. Hankoff, and Bernard Rosen who participated in this research.

This work was supported by Public Health Service Grant MH 0 1983 and MH 0 5090 from the National Institute of Mental Health.

ment was concise minimal psychotherapeutic management. The Engel-hardt-Margolis investigation took place over a number of years and had a large population; Rothman's was shorter and had a small sample, yet resulted in statistically significant findings. Both studies need to be elaborated and replicated. The deeper understanding of psychopathology, subtypes of patients, and the variables associated with drugs, doctor, family, and community-treatment milieu demonstrate the complexity of the problems and the need for devising new methods for exploring them.

Until very recently, hospitalization has been the community's principal approach toward combating the disruptive symptomatology and social handicaps of seriously ill schizophrenic patients. Unlike the procedure in other illnesses, in schizophrenia the decision to hospitalize has been in most instances the family's, with the physician acting as "midwife" at the moment of hospitalization. Only during the past few years have alternative modes of dealing with the schizophrenic patient been considered. These alternative approaches might be characterized as follows: substitution, when necessary, of frequent brief hospitalizations in place of the heretofore "popular" chronic institutionalization; development of community-based mental health centers offering comprehensive care and treatment; and large-scale use of psychoactive drugs as a therapeutic modality. The goal of maintaining the schizophrenic patient in the community has been accepted in principle by many state and local mental health departments and is finding support from an increasing number of psychiatric practitioners.

The revolution in patient care represented by the concept of a comprehensive, community-based psychiatric treatment service is the consequence of another revolution—the psychopharmacologic revolution. *Availability of drugs capable of modifying the symptoms of schizophrenic patients has given rise to the hope that large numbers of psychotic patients might be treated on an outpatient basis at relatively low cost in money and professional manpower.*

In 1957, the Psychopharmacology Treatment and Research Unit of the Downstate Medical Center undertook a large-scale research program involving treatment and maintenance of a considerable group of schizophrenic patients within the Brooklyn community. The program was established at a free public clinic and is an active community project. Treatment consisted of the use of phenothiazine agents combined with minimal supportive psychotherapy. The availability of an objective quantifiable treatment input—ie, the psychotropic drug—encouraged the Unit to undertake a systematic placebo-controlled long-term study.

Our patient population was drawn primarily from the intake of the Mental Health Clinic of the Kings County Hospital Center, Brooklyn, New York. The population represented a cross section of ambulatory schizophrenic patients; included were males and females between the ages of 18 and 44, with a mean age of 30. All patients had a primary diagnosis of schizophrenia with evidence of having been ill for at least one year. Approximately 25% of our patients were Negro. Over half our patients had not completed high school, and the majority fell into Hollingshead's Social Classes 4 and 5, representing the lower socio-economic groups.

Whereas our population was clearly schizophrenic and also not acute, the patients varied considerably in degree of chronicity and history of previous treatment. More than 50% had been ill ten years or more. Ten percent had never received any psychiatric treatment prior to admission to our clinic. Another 10% had received only outpatient treatment. Thirty percent had been hospitalized less than 90 days in aggregate prior to admission. Only 25% had experienced an aggregate amount of hospitalization in excess of 12 months prior to admission to our clinic. *Thus our patients, though essentially chronic in duration of illness, varied considerably in amount of previous hospitalization. Approximately 50% of our patients had maintained an essentially ambulatory status prior to clinic admission.*

Between 1957 and 1963, over 750 patients were admitted to our Unit. For research purposes the sample was divided into two parts. The first 500 patients—admitted between March 1, 1958, and December 31, 1961—were designated as our basic research population. The remaining 250 patients, admitted under identical intake criteria and exposed to identical treatment conditions, were designated as our replication sample for the purpose of validating findings on the first 500 patients.

Treatment procedures and research design have been presented in detail previously in publications.[1-4] Upon admission to the clinic, patients were randomly assigned to chlorpromazine (Thorazine), promazine (Sparine), or placebo, and remained on the same medication during the entire period of clinic attendance. Medication was administered under double-blind conditions in the form of identical capsules. The treating psychiatrists were not aware of the identity of the medication a patient received, but they were aware of the identity of the three agents used. The psychiatrists were free to vary the dose according to their clinical judgment. The mean dose for the active agents was approximately 200 mg daily; for placebo the equivalent of 350 mg daily was prescribed.

Clinic visits were scheduled weekly for the first month, biweekly for the next two months, and monthly thereafter. Information about the patient's home and community functioning was obtained on a monthly basis from a reliable relative. Patients were free to leave the clinic at will, no attempt being made to "force" them back into treatment. Under these conditions, dropout rates from treatment proved to be considerable. The two primary sources of dropouts were "hospitalization" and "spontaneous dropout." The term "hospitalization" as used here refers to hospitalizations occurring during the course of the patient's treatment at our clinic. The fate of the "spontaneous dropouts" was not known to us. For the purpose of this presentation, these patients are considered "not hospitalized."

In our 1960 first report[1] on the prevention of hospitalization of schizophrenic outpatients, we introduced our findings with the following statement:

> The dramatic effects and the value of ataractic agents in psychiatric treatment have by now become a clinically accepted fact. It remains for psychopharmacologic research to validate the broad lines laid down by clinical findings. *One major area in need of objective validation is the effect of therapy with ataractic drugs on the hospitalization rate among psychiatric patients prone to breakdown. It is obviously of great importance whether the new drugs are able to reduce the hospitalization rate among patients with the major psychiatric illnesses.* Although several clinical and statistical reports claim that ataractic treatment prevents hospitalization, a review of the literature fails to reveal a controlled study verifying this proposition.

Our findings strikingly demonstrated the effectiveness of psychoactive drugs in the prevention of hospitalization among schizophrenic outpatients. During the first 18 months of the research clinic's operation, of 56 patients treated with placebo, 28.5% had been hospitalized, as opposed to only 4.8% of 62 patients treated with chlorpromazine ($\chi^2 = 12.27$, d.f. $= 1$, P <0.001). The hospitalization rate under promazine treatment fell between that under chlorpromazine and under placebo. Of 55 patients treated with promazine, 18.2% were hospitalized. The difference between chlorpromazine and promazine was significant at the .05 level. The overall hospitalization rate for the entire cohort of 173 patients was 16.7%. The significantly lower hospitalization rate with chlorpromazine treatment was sustained when the patient subgroups were equated for ratings relative to history of previous hospitalization and severity of illness. Spontaneous dropout from treatment (a major source of sample attrition other than hospitalization) did not prove to be a confounding factor; spontaneous dropouts from the three treatment groups were placebo, 33.9%; promazine, 34.5%; and chlorpromazine, 40.3%.

Throughout succeeding months, we realized that duration of treatment exposure was an important factor affecting rate of hospitalization. When we again examined hospitalization rates among our patients in 1963, now on a sample of 445 consecutive admissions,[2] our 1960 findings were not duplicated, as can be observed in Table 1. Of 142 patients treated with placebo 29.6% were hospitalized, a

TABLE 1

**Comparison of Hospitalization Rates by Drug Treatment
1960 and 1963 Samples**

Drug	1960		1963	
	Number	%	Number	%
Placebo	16	28.6	42	29.6
Promazine	10	18.2	42	28.0
Chlorpromazine	3	4.8	29	19.0
Total	29	16.7	113	25.4

figure essentially not different from that obtained in 1960. However, of 150 patients treated with promazine, 28.0% were hospitalized, and of 153 patients treated with chlorpromazine, 19.0% were hospitalized. Chlorpromazine remained superior to placebo in its lesser hospitalization rate ($\chi^2 = 4.55$, $P < 0.05$), but clearly the superiority over placebo was considerably less impressive than reported in 1960. A comparison of hospitalization rates between chlorpromazine and promazine no longer yielded a significant difference. The overall hospitalization rate in 1963 was 25.4%, a considerable rise when compared with that reported in 1960 (16.7%).

We attributed this rise in hospitalization rate to differences in duration of treatment exposure. Whereas minimum and maximum duration of treatment exposure of the 1960 sample was one and 18 months respectively, exposure of the 1963 sample was 15 and 61 months. Obviously, patients in the 1963 sample had considerably more opportunity to be hospitalized than the patients in the 1960 sample.

To test this assumption, the hospitalization rates for the 1960 sample were reexamined as of 1963, with the minimum treatment exposure increased to 43 months and the maximum to 61 months. The results of this anlysis, as shown in Table 2, revealed that of the

TABLE 2

Hospitalization Rates of the 1960 Sample by Drug Treatment in 1960 and 1963

Drug	1960 Analysis		1963 Analysis	
	Number	%	Number	%
Placebo (N = 56)	16	28.6	18	32.1
Promazine (N = 55)	10	18.2	15	27.3
Chlorpromazine (N = 62)	3	4.8	9	14.5
Total (N = 173)	29	16.7	42	24.2

56 patients treated with placebo, 32.1% were hospitalized; of 55 patients treated with promazine, 27.3% were hospitalized; and of 62 patients treated with chlorpromazine, 14.5% were hospitalized. The overall hospitalization rate was 24.2%. Statistically, the findings had the same significance as the larger 1963 sample. Duration of treatment exposure was a significant factor influencing treatment outcome—first, by influencing overall hospitalization rates (comparing 1960 and 1963, 16.7% versus 25.4%); and second, by demonstrating differential effects in hospitalization rates by treatment. Although the number of patients hospitalized on placebo remained relatively constant, the number of patients hospitalized on drugs rose precipitously.

The findings suggested that the effect of phenothiazines on hospitalization rates was short-term. It was possible to demonstrate that during the first six months of treatment exposure, the hospitalization rate for chlorpromazine (8.5%) was significantly lower (P<.01) than that for placebo (21.1%).[3] The rate for promazine (14.4%) was not differentiable from the other two. During the second six months of treatment the rates for the three treatments were statistically indistinguishable: placebo 16.0%, promazine 10.1%, and chlor-promazine 11.0%.

When analysis of hospitalization was continued beyond one year, a very different picture emerged. The hospitalization rate for placebo dropped to zero and the rates for both phenothiazine treatments (chlorpromazine 9.2%, promazine 20.0%) were significantly higher. The short-term effect was certainly confirmed. The progressive increase in hospitalization rates among drug-treated patients versus time raised the question as to whether and when the hospitalization of the phenothiazine-treated patients would equal that of the placebo-treated patients. The data seemed so orderly that we boldly extrapolated the phenothiazine curves, and predicted that this would occur when patients had an opportunity to be in treatment for a minimum of 17 months under promazine and 30 months under chlorpromazine.

In January 1967,[4] we reported on the hospitalization rates of our three drug groups after an additional 35 months of treatment exposure, hospitalization rates being determined as of March 1, 1966. Since no new patients were admitted to the study after December 31, 1961, all patients had the opportunity of remaining in treatment at least 50 months before hospitalization rates were determined. Figure 1 taken from this report shows the cumulative rate of hospitalization by drug treatment for successive three-month periods of treatment exposure up to 48 months. The total rate after 48 months is also presented.

Inspection of the curves reveals that during the first six months the placebo rate is higher and decreases less than that of either promazine or chlorpromazine. During the second six months the rate of increase of the placebo curve declines and becomes comparable to the rate of increase of the other two curves. Between 12 and 18 months the rate of increase of the placebo curve further declines, becoming lower than that of either of the phenothiazine-treated groups. After 18 months the rates of increase of the three curves are comparable. Thus, following 12 months of placebo treatment and 18 months of drug treatment, a plateau is reached and few additional hospitalizations occur. Of a total of 45 hospitalizations on placebo, 42 occurred in the first 12 months, one after 29 months, one at 39 months, and one at 51 months.

The constancy of the placebo hospitalization rate beyond 12 months suggested that in our group of schizophrenic patients only a limited and a stable finite number were prone to hospitalization.

Fig. 1: Cumulative Hospitalization Rates by Drug Treatment*

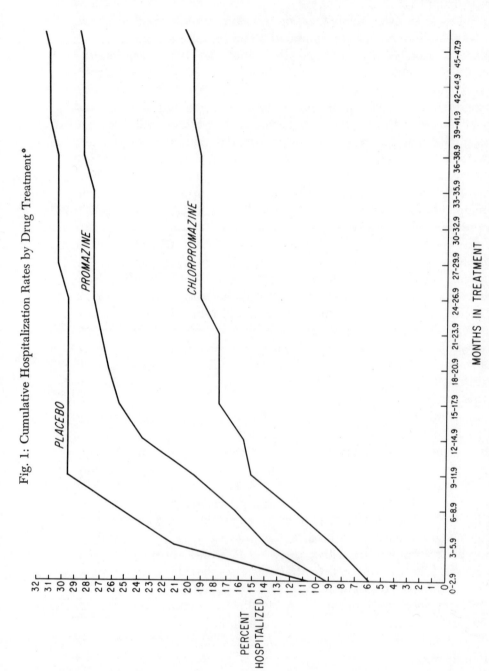

* Previously published in *Archives of General Psychiatry*, vol 16, Jan 1967. Reprinted with permission.

The constancy of the hospitalization rate attributable to placebo treatment was further confirmed by a review of the literature.[2] Therefore, in making statistical evaluations of rates of hospitalization at 12 months of treatment and beyond, we used the 12-month placebo rate (29.6%) as our expected frequency. This is in contrast to the usual procedure of testing independence of all samples from their common mean. We felt further justified in this procedure in view of the relatively large size ($N = 142$) of the placebo group.

A statistical comparison was made of the cumulative hospitalization rates for some of the successive periods of treatment exposure shown in Figure 1. After 12 months of treatment exposure, hospitalization rates for chlorpromazine (15.1%) and promazine (19.7%) are significantly lower than the rate of the placebo-treated patients (29.6%)—chlorpromazine, $x^2 = 15.28$, P<0.001; promazine, $x^2 = 7.10$, P<0.01. By 15 months the promazine hospitalization rate (23.7%) is statistically comparable to that of placebo (29.6%), and remains so thereafter. However, even at 48 months the chlorpromazine hospitalization rate (19.7%) remains significantly lower than that of placebo (29.6%)—$x^2 = 7.10$, P<0.01.

We had previously expressed concern whether the reduction of hospitalization under chlorpromazine treatment represented "delay" or "prevention" of hospitalization.[2, 3] The data in Figure 1 clearly suggest that chlorpromazine treatment significantly alters and reduces the risk of hospitalization among our schizophrenic outpatients. To conclude that the action of chlorpromazine is one of prevention requires, however, the assumption that patients hospitalized while treated with different agents are similar in terms of hospitalization proneness. Impressed as we were with the effectiveness of chlorpromazine, we could not ignore the observation that apparently not all schizophrenic patients were vulnerable to hospitalization, since only a subgroup of approximately 30% were hospitalized.

The assumption that among a group of schizophrenic outpatients only a finite portion is prone to hospitalization is of course clinically quite tenable. Schizophrenic patients are not alike. The term "schizophrenic" includes many classes of patients, differing in chronicity, severity of illness, and in the quantity and quality of their presenting symptomatology. This is particularly true of an outpatient population. The ability of the ambulatory schizophrenic to maintain outpatient adjustment is the result of a complex of factors, including at the minimum: (1) the patient's symptomatology; (2) the family's and/or the community's tolerance for the patient's deviance; and (3) the patient's "tolerance" for his own symptomatology, in the sense that the presence of a relatively high level of psychotic symptomatology does not prevent him from maintaining his social role and usual functions without too much resultant trouble with his environment.

Despite our evidence in support of a finite subgroup of hospitalization-prone patients, the identification of the *prone* and *non-prone* patient posed complex problems. Reviewers of literature dealing with the clinical course of schizophrenic patients[5-7] were generally agreed on the paucity of definitive findings. We approached the problem of prediction of hospitalization by studying and comparing our hospitalized and not-hospitalized placebo-treated patients. We had a considerable body of biographic, social, psychologic, and psychiatric data, which we obtained on each patient at intake into our clinic. We did not have to rely on retrospective data, and we had over 140 placebo-treated patients to use as a pool in order to construct a scale to predict hospitalization proneness (HPS).[8] The component items of the final scale, together with the criteria for scoring, are presented in Table 3. Variables were scored so that a high HPS score represents the *non-prone*, and a low score represents the *prone* end of the continuum. Scores range from 0 to 11.

In order to classify patients as either *prone* or *non-prone*, it was necessary to determine that point in the distribution of HPS scores that would most effectively differentiate hospitalized from non-hospitalized patients. To establish this dichotomy, a comparison was made of the distribution of the HPS scores obtained by the hospitalized and non-hospitalized placebo-treated patients used to develop this scale. On the basis of this comparison, the *prone* patient was defined as one with an HPS score of 6.0 or less; the *non-prone* patient was defined as one with an HPS score of 6.5 or more. This method of classification was used throughout this study. The final scale consisted of eight variables drawn from only three of the sources available: psychologic, social behavioral, and biographic.

The *prone* patient can be described as (*a*) reflecting a poor capacity to organize and synthesize experience (low F+%); (*b*) having a low level of social adaptability and intelligence (Low Porteus Maze Quantitative Score);[9, 10] (*c*) having an undifferentiated perception of social roles (in TAT stories); and (*d*) having a low level of manifest anxiety.[11] In terms of his social behavior, the

TABLE 3

Components of the Hospitalization Proneness Scale (HPS)*

	PRONE		NON-PRONE	
Variable	Score	Weight	Score	Weight
Psychological				
Rorschach F+%	00–79	0	80+	1
Porteus-Maze:				
Quantitative Score	00–12.5	0	13+	1
TAT Role Perception	00–10	0	11+	1
Manifest Anxiety Scale	00–10	0	11+	1
Social Behavior				
Explicit Oppositionalism	00.0–16.9	0	17.0+	3
Solitariness	24.6+	0	00.0–24.5	2
Biographical				
Months in Previous Psychiatric				
Treatment	12+	0	00–11.9	1
Index of Social Position	62+	0	00–61	1

* Previously published in *Journal of Abnormal Psychology*, vol. 72, no. 6, and reproduced by permission.

prone patient was described by a close relative as being low in explicit oppositionalism and high in solitariness. In addition, he had a low index of social position, defined by his educational and occupational attainment,[12] and had been in psychiatric treatment a cumulative total of one year or longer prior to admission to our clinic. It is of interest to note that none of the psychiatric variables defining the patient's nosology or salient symptom picture—ie, the degree of paranoid or schizophrenic thought disorder, hallucinations, or delusions—was significantly related to future hospitalization.

Table 4 presents the data indicating the ability of the HPS to differentiate hospitalized from non-hospitalized patients in the original placebo-treated group. As Table 4 indicates, the HPS is clearly linked to the incidence of hospitalization in this group of schizophrenic outpatients. As would be expected, significantly more *prone* patients (42 or 48.8%) were hospitalized during the course of treatment as compared to the *non-prone* group (3 or 5.4%)—$\chi^2 = 29.62$, P<.001.

Table 4 also presents the relationship between the HPS and hospitalization among placebo-treated patients in our cross-validation sample. The results for this group are consistent with those

TABLE 4

**Hospitalization Rate by HPS Group in Original and
Cross-Validation Placebo Samples**

Original Sample

HPS Group	HOSPITALIZED		NOT-HOSPITALIZED	
	Number	%	Number	%
Prone (N = 86)	42	48.8	44	51.2
Non-Prone (N = 56)	3	5.4	53	94.6
Total (N = 142)	45	31.7	97	68.3

$X^2 = 29.62$, d.f. $= 1$, $\rho < .001$

Cross-Validation Sample

HPS Group	HOSPITALIZED		NOT-HOSPITALIZED	
Prone (N = 26)	16	61.5	10	38.5
Non-Prone (N = 13)	1	7.7	12	92.3
Total (N = 39)	17	43.6	22	56.4

$X^2 = 10.22$, d.f. $= 1$, $\rho < .01$

presented above. Again, significantly more *prone* patients were hospitalized (16 or 61.5%) than *non-prone* (1 or 7.7%)—$\chi^2 = 10.22$, P<.01.

In comparing the results of the original and cross-validation placebo samples the similarity in hospitalization rates for both *prone* and *non-prone* patients is apparent. Thus, we found that not only was it possible to replicate the original results with an independent sample under identical treatment conditions, but also that there was no loss of predictive power.

Development of the Hospitalization Proneness Scale (HPS) permitted us to study the effects of our two drug treatments separately for *prone* and *non-prone* patients. In Figures 2 and 3 we have plotted the cumulative hospitalization rates for *prone* and *non-prone* patients separately for each treatment condition. The method of constructing the HPS dictated that there would be a maximal differentiation of the rates for the placebo-treated *prone* and *non-prone* groups. Fifty-seven months after admission of the last patient in the cohort, the rate of hospitalization for placebo-treated *prone* patients was 50% and only 5.4% for placebo-treated *non-prone* patients.

The effect of phenothiazines on the hospitalization rate of *prone*

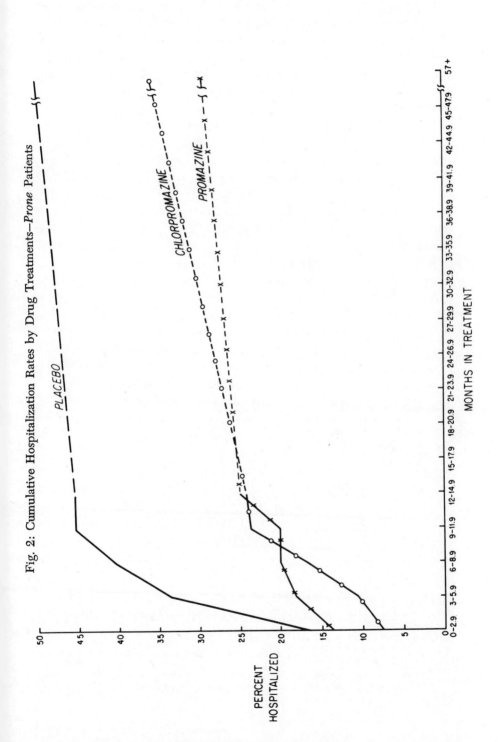

Fig. 2: Cumulative Hospitalization Rates by Drug Treatments—*Prone* Patients

patients is clear. Both chlorpromazine (N = 70) and promazine (N = 85) have significantly lower rates of hospitalization than placebo after 57 months (chlorpromazine 35.7%, promazine 29.4%, placebo 50%.)* The shapes of the placebo and chlorpromazine curves are very similar to those presented in Figure 1. The shape of the promazine curve has considerably flattened and shifted away from the placebo curve toward the chlorpromazine curve.

This shift in the promazine curve foreshadows the findings for the *non-prone* patients shown in Figure 3. Here it can be observed that the hospitalization rates for placebo and chlorpromazine (N = 82) start and remain low, and are not significantly different from each other. However, the rate for promazine (N = 67) rises rather rapidly during the first 12 months of treatment, and reaches a plateau after approximately 15 months. The rate for promazine is significantly greater than those of the other treatments after 57 months.† Thus promazine, in contrast to chlorpromazine and placebo, has a seemingly negative effect among *non-prone* patients.

An interesting finding made during the development of the HPS is the lack of relationship between hospitalization and either psychopathologic manifestations at intake or nosologic subgroups. In relation to psychopathology, it is important to distinguish its role as a *predictor* (representing the potential for hospitalization) from that of a *precipitant* (leading to the actual occurrence of the event). Although psychopathology may be irrelevant as a predictor of hospitalization, as our study would suggest, a sudden upsurge in symptom level just prior to hospitalization may be relevant to the decision to hospitalize. Thus, psychopathology may be important in the role of a concomitant treatment event. Drug dose and the emergence of somatic side effects could be other such factors that play a role in precipitating hospitalization.

Examining the life histories of our patients at the time they entered our clinic, we found that 80% had experienced at least one brief hospitalization prior to admission to the clinic. Observing the fate of those patients who remained with us for treatment, we find on an overall basis that under placebo treatment only 30% became hospitalized. This suggests that drug treatment is only one factor

* Promazine versus placebo, $\chi^2 = 7.56$, d.f. = 1, P < .005; chlorpromazine versus placebo, $\chi^2 = 3.20$, d.f. = 1, P < .05. Since these were one-sided hypotheses, one-tailed tests of significance were used.

† Promazine versus placebo, $\chi^2 = 10.99$, d.f. = 1, P < .005, one-tailed test as previously indicated. Promazine versus chlorpromazine, $\chi^2 = 7.87$, d.f. = 1, P < .01, two-tailed test.

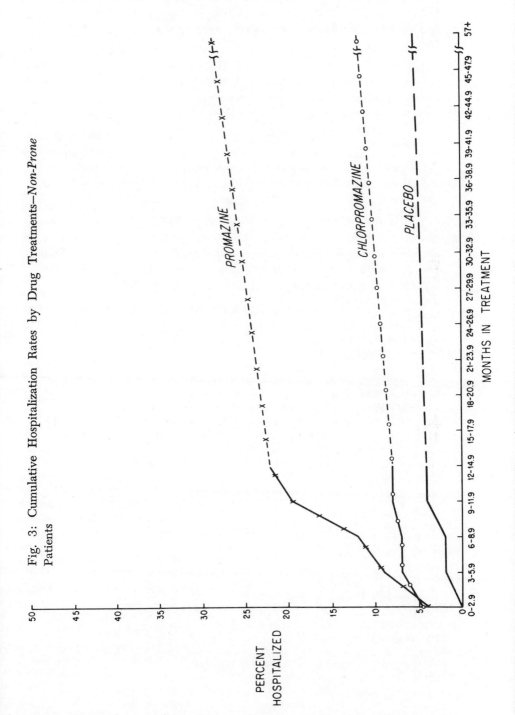

Fig. 3: Cumulative Hospitalization Rates by Drug Treatments—*Non-Prone* Patients

influencing reduction in hospitalization among our schizophrenic outpatients. The difference in overall hospitalization rates in our clinic population before and after admission to the clinic calls attention to the important contribution of the doctor and the clinic milieu to the prevention of hospitalization among our patients.

In summary: We have presented evidence that drugs, especially chlorpromazine, are effective in altering both the timing and rate of hospitalization in chronic schizophrenic outpatients. The Hospitalization Proneness Scale (HPS) has proved a valuable research tool. By identifying the *prone* and *non-prone* patient we were able to establish differential drug effects for these two populations. We were also able to identify positive and negative drug effects.

Our findings attest to the fact that research still needs to be done. We know relatively little as to how phenothiazines and other drugs mediate both desired and undesired changes. We need to know much more about the hospitalization process, particularly as it operates at the family level: *who* gets hospitalized, *by whom, when,* and *for what reason.* Perhaps when we learn more about these aspects we may succeed in developing more effective drugs and treatment plans for preventing hospitalization among schizophrenic patients.

REFERENCES

1. Engelhardt, D. M., Freedman, N., Glick, B. S., Hankoff, L. D., Mann, D., and Margolis, R.: Prevention of Psychiatric Hospitalization with Use of Psychopharmacological Agents, *JAMA*, 173:147–149, 1960.
2. Engelhardt, D. M., Rosen, B., Freedman, N., Mann, D., and Margolis, R.: Phenothiazines in Prevention of Psychiatric Hospitalization: II. Duration of Treatment Exposure, *JAMA*, 186:981–983, 1963.
3. Engelhardt, D. M., Freedman, N., Rosen, B., Mann, D., and Margolis, R.: Phenothiazines in Prevention of Psychiatric Hospitalization: III. Prevention or Delay of Hospitalization, *Arch. Gen. Psychiat.*, 11:162–169, 1964.
4. Engelhardt, D. M., Rosen, B., Freedman, N., and Margolis, R.: Phenothiazines in Prevention of Psychiatric Hospitalization: IV. Delay or Prevention of Hospitalization: A Reevaluation, *Arch. Gen. Psychiat.*, 16, 98–102, 1967.
5. Windle, C.: Psychological Tests in Psychopathological Prognosis, *Psychol. Bull.*, 49, 451–482, 1952.
6. Zubin, J., and Windle, C.: Psychological Prognosis of Outcome in Mental Disorders, *J. Abnorm. Soc. Psychol.*, 49, 272–281, 1954.
7. Huston, P. E., and Pepernick, N. C.: "Prognosis in Schizophrenia," in L. Bellak (ed.): *Schizophrenia*, New York: Logos, 1958, pp. 531–546.
8. Freedman, N., Rosen, B., Engelhardt, D. M., and Margolis, R. A.: Prediction of Psychiatric Hospitalization: I. Measurement of Hospitalization Proneness, *J. Abnorm. Psych.*, 72: 6, 468–477, December 1967.

9. Porteus, S. D.: *Porteus Maze Test and Intelligence*, Palo Alto, Calif.: Pacific Books, 1950.
10. Porteus, S. D.: *Maze Test Recent Advances*, Palo Alto, Calif.: Pacific Books, 1955.
11. Benig, A. W.: Development of Short Form of Manifest Anxiety Scale, *J. Consult. Psychol.*, 20, 384, 1956.
12. Hollingshead, A. B., and Redlich, F. C.: *Social Class and Mental Illness*, New York: John Wiley & Sons, 1958.

7

Comparing Therapeutic Results
of Community Care
in Early Schizophrenics*

by THEODORE ROTHMAN†

Rothman and his group investigated a cohort of first-admission, early, acute schizophrenics, with specific criteria, from their admission to Camarillo State Hospital until their discharge into the Los Angeles community. This cohort was followed through their trials and tribulations, the experiment having been designed to compare a variety of treatments for their community aftercare. It was found that this subtype of early, acute schizophrenic patient, if quickly removed from the state hospital milieu, rarely needs to be rehospitalized. It also was discovered that the patient generally functioned well and quickly in community life and that he could manage successfully without drugs or intensive psychotherapy. Concise minimal psychotherapeutic management seemed to be the treatment of choice for this group.

The numbers of patients and length of follow-up were too small to make

* This study was done at the Los Angeles State Mental Hygiene Clinic of the State of California Department of Mental Hygiene in collaboration with Camarillo State Hospital as an Early Clinical Drug Evaluation Unit (ECDEU) of the Psychopharmacology Research Branch of the National Institute of Mental Health: supported by PHS Grant MH 11725-01; a grant-in-aid from the Albert A. Epstein Fund of the Rush Research Foundation and from Sandoz Pharmaceutical Company. Computing assistance was obtained from the Health Sciences Computing Facility, University of California at Los Angeles, sponsored by National Institute of Health Grant FR-3.

† The author gratefully acknowledges the following as having actively collaborated in this study: M. H. Firestone, M.D., Associate to the Principal Investigator; H. Austin, MSW; S. Conrad, M.D.; A. Darbonne, Ph.D.; N. Dugan, M.D.; E. Kris, M.D.; A. LaPolla, M.D.; and the late Louis R. Nash, M.D. Also assisting in this study were Wilfrid Dixon, Ph.D., and Lee H. Youkeles, M.S., of the Health Sciences Computing Facility, UCLA.

*a strong case for what was called "contemporary moral therapy." Although
the sample was not sufficiently large to make wide generalizations, statistical significance for this group was quite high. Thus, it is believed that
a sufficiently large number should be further studied and followed for a
longer period of time. The indications are strong that future results might
very well resemble the conclusions reached in this study. The important
aspect of this investigation is the possibility that relatively simple, meaningful psychiatric management of a large majority of early, acute schizophrenic patients may successfully be carried out in the community, with
uncomplicated, brief, inexpensive aftercare treatment.*

Although much enthusiasm has been generated, there have been no
rigorously controlled studies reported that demonstrate the efficacy
of the facilities exemplifying the community mental health center
as defined by federal regulations.[1] The problems associated with
establishing such facilities have not been sufficiently defined. Similarly, adequate preparations have not been made for the patients'
reintegration into the community.[2]

The contemporary model of a mental hospital and its ancillary
facilities, called the mental health center approach, had its beginnings in moral treatment of the mentally ill as derived from the 18th
and 19th centuries. [3-7] In the mental health center, the contemporary concept of moral treatment has been conjoined with the public
health and welfare state, social and political models. Even though
this approach opens many new doors to opportunities for treatment,
its novelty makes it most difficult to collect reliable data concerning
these programs.[8]

Though the new moral humanitarian aspects of the local community mental hospital and the ancillary aftercare services seem to
be of considerable merit, compared to the previous custodialism, the
programs now hastily activated appear to offer completely new
medical, social, and political programs. There is a most urgent need,
therefore, to evaluate a number of aspects of these new mental
health programs with better scientific methods.[10, 11]

Several projects have been undertaken that have focused on drugs
and community care.[9-11] Greenblatt[12] and others have performed
clinical studies and published discussions involving patients in a
variety of transitional facilities after hospitalization. Experience

with management of major mental illness in the community has been described by Epps and Zusman.[13, 14] In the United Kingdom, Sainsbury and Grad[15] made an attempt to compare the patients treated with community services—eg, outpatient clinics, day hospitals, and home services—with those treated in mental hospitals, the conclusion being reached that community care is a feasible type of management. They, as well as Pasamanick[16] in his tests and Friedman[17, 18] in his project, were able to treat the patient effectively in his home by using psychoactive drugs and ancillary aids. Similarly, Friedman demonstrated that it was possible to achieve encouraging results in the management of home cases through psychiatric and community services by using a combination of these services with psychoactive drugs.

Preliminary studies of the State of California Day Treatment Centers have been carried out by Dondis[19] and McMillan and Dondis.[20] More recently, Kris[21] has shown that aftercare clinics in the State of New York using psychoactive drugs and other therapies are effective in maintaining the patient in the community, thus preventing hospitalization. Kris also has demonstrated that the relapsed schizophrenics admitted to a day hospital in New York State spend much less treatment time there before discharge than if they had been hospitalized.

However, one of our pilot studies performed at the State of California Los Angeles Day Treatment Center[22] has led us to believe that many patients may be managed as effectively and with less dependency by more concise minimal treatment than that presently received.

A number of recent studies on schizophrenic inpatients demonstrated that psychoactive drugs and the current form of moral treatment interacted.[23, 24] Greenblatt[25] and others have further shown that social therapy and psychoactive drugs combined complement each other in the treatment of the patient from the hospital to the community. The interaction of combined treatments was further confirmed by Engelhardt's[26-29] aftercare studies on the prevention of hospitalization with psychopharmacologic agents. He presents controlled evidence that minimal psychotherapy and psychoactive drugs, especially chlorpromazine, are effective in altering both the time-length and rate of hospitalization in chronic schizophrenics. By identifying the hospital-prone patient he is able to establish differential drug effects. He concludes that psychoactive drugs are one of the significant factors influencing reduction in hospitalization of schizophrenic patients; other factors include the relationship with the doctor, and the clinic milieu.

Since it is believed that the aftercare facility, and its contemporary form of moral treatment, plays a crucial role in the reintegration of the patient and in helping to sustain him in the community, it is imperative that the specific therapeutic factors involved in the management of these patients be clearly and carefully identified.

Our general aim relative to the study described in this chapter was to ascertain how to perform a valid controlled project under difficult conditions with a cohort of early acute schizophrenic patients, studying them from their first hospitalization to their aftercare in the community and their subsequent patterns of reintegration. Our secondary aim was to measure the effect of the patient on the community, the family, the physician, and his treatment.

In order to accomplish our aims, a number of different psychiatric approaches were compared: first, effect of maximal versus minimal psychiatric management; second, a double-blind investigation of drug versus placebo; and third, a study of the influence of non-pharmacologic factors (the role of the doctor, family, and milieu), which we shall call modified moral treatment. To further delineate our findings, we measured the effect of different psychiatric management on socialization; recreational activity; employment; and contention in the conjugal and lineal family.

METHODS AND PROCEDURES

1. Criteria for Selection of Patients

Patients were selected and followed through the course of their illness at the State of California Camarillo State Hospital. Selection was made by the hospital staff and research social worker (RSW). Patients were brought to the attention of the RSW from the State of California Los Angeles Mental Hygiene Clinic (LASMHC) Early Clinic Evaluation Unit (ECDEU) by the state hospital physicians.

Patients selected had the following criteria: stratification of males and females; age 20 to 50 years; normal intelligence; early acute schizophrenia with symptoms present of at least three of the following: thinking disorder, hallucinations, delusions, disorientation, catatonic motor disturbance, disturbance of affect (inappropriateness, anhedonia, flatness of effect), severe disturbance of social interaction; first hospital admission with hospital stay of not longer than six months; and a history of schizophrenia of less than 18 months. The duration of illness was measured from the time of severe malfunctioning on social, vocational, interpersonal, and educational levels and three severe symptoms of schizophrenia as defined above.

The patient lived in the metropolitan area with reasonably available transportation. He had a home or its alternate available to him and a significant person or persons serving as a reference group. Excluded from the study were imminently suicidal or homicidal persons judged in terms of the present; all severe illnesses, especially cardiac, renal, hematopoietic, or liver dysfunction; all chronic alcoholics, drug addicts, sociopaths, and brain syndromes. The patients' primary mode of communication was English.

2. Procedures

Our RSW was in part stationed at Camarillo State Hospital. The patient's hospital folder contained a sheet designating him as a research patient for the project chosen by the hospital staff and the RSW. This "flagged" the patient so that we could follow him throughout his stay at the hospital. A few days before the patient was placed on home leave, the RSW was contacted. There was continued communication between the RSW of the LASMHC until his departure from the state hospital and release to the LASMHC. One or two weeks before discharge the RSW informed the LASMHC and received a code number for the patient, as well as an appointment with a specific psychiatrist.

3. Admission to LASMHC (ECDEU)

The patient became a regular patient of the LASMHC after his release from the state hospital.[30] He had a prearranged appointment with a specific physician, as determined by our preplanned design. The treating physician informed the patient on admission that he was part of a special treatment group and that it was important for him to take his medication and his tests and keep his appointments, to complete his treatment successfully. The treating physician was informed whether the patient was on maximal or minimal treatment.

During the first week, the following tests were performed at the clinic: Brief Psychiatric Rating Scale (BPRS) and the Community Resources Check List (CRCL) indicating the community services suggested to the RSW for aiding the patient. These included socialization, education, vocation, financial, family relations (placement or treatment of child or other family members), religion (pastoral guidance, etc.), legal (aid concerning legal problems), physical status (medical, dental), patient's living quarters, and miscellaneous suggestions. NIMH, HEW, Drug Study Form was filled out.

4. Treatment

Eighty patients were selected from Camarillo State Hospital for this experiment; for various reasons, 20 of these patients never arrived. Sixty came to the LASMHC, and each patient was placed in one of four treatment plans in a balanced design. The BPRS was done on admission during the test week.

TREATMENT PLAN I. Maximal psychiatric management plus thioridazine (Mellaril): dosage mean, 400 mg/daily.

TREATMENT PLAN II. Maximal psychiatric management plus placebo: dosage mean, 4 capsules placebo/daily.

TREATMENT PLAN III. Concise minimal psychiatric management plus thioridazine (Mellaril): dosage mean, 400 mg/daily.

TREATMENT PLAN IV. Concise minimal psychiatric management plus placebo: dosage mean, 4 capsules placebo/daily.

To further define our methods of treatment—*maximal psychiatric management* consisted of individual and group psychotherapy, with respectively at least one one hour weekly, and was augmented by a schedule of planned rehabilitation utilizing community services for social, spiritual, educational, recreational, and vocational therapy combined with either drug or placebo. *Concise minimal psychiatric management* consisted of a weekly brief psychotherapeutic interview of not more than 15 minutes structured to meet the emergency needs of the patient, in combination with either drug or placebo. Social service when absolutely necessary was given.

After the third, sixth, and twelfth week, a BPRS was done by the treating psychiatrist and two other nontreating psychiatrists rating individually, involving the same patients by the same psychiatrists.

The RSW visited the home on admission to ECDEU and between the third, sixth, and twelfth week, a Home Visit Rating Scale (HVRS) being performed on each occasion. Follow-up was conducted throughout the project; and HVRS was done every three months.

All patients who cooperated for three weeks of treatment were considered part of the project. If a patient appeared to be an imminent dropout, the BPRS and the HVRS were recorded. Reason for dropout was ascertained whenever possible.

Drug Schedule

Thioridazine (Mellaril) and placebo were administered in No. 2 pink capsules, each containing 100 mg of thioridazine (Mellaril) or an inert compound (placebo). The ECDEU staff were "blind" as to whether those on Treatment Plans I to IV were receiving the psychoactive drug or placebo.

Whenever possible, we attempted to maintain dose levels at 300 to 400 mg daily. The standard procedure was left to the treating physician's discretion, according to the patient's presumed response to the therapeutic procedure. Similarly, we attempted to prescribe a similar number of placebo capsules.

Duration of drug treatment was 12 weeks; a minimum of six weeks was maintained for evaluation and analysis for this study. Since some of the patients selected were on drug treatment at the hospital immediately prior to admission to this study, the first week was utilized for withdrawal of the drug, during which time placebo was administered. No longer than two weeks was allowed for drug withdrawal of these patients.

Laboratory Examinations

Thioridazine (Mellaril) is believed to be a well-tried psychoactive agent, relatively free of side effects when taken in our prescribed dose. Laboratory procedures could be performed when warranted, but only when side effects occurred.

Documentation of Psychological and Social Assessment

1. NIMH, HEW Drug Study Form was administered on admissions to the ECDEU project and was to be filled out during the entire study involving social, psychiatric, and medical history and changes of psychopharmacology—the side effects, laboratory tests, and global evaluation—and the results during the entire clinical trial.

2. Brief Psychiatric Rating Scale (BPRS)* was done on admittance, the third, sixth, and twelfth weeks of the clinical trial, and a follow-up was done by the treating psychiatrist and the two non-treating psychiatrists simultaneously.

3. Home Visit Rating Scale (HVRS).† This test was done as long

* Overall and Gorham modified by Rothman et al.
† Rothman, Austin.

as a week or two after admission and around the third, sixth, and twelfth weeks, at follow-up approximately the same week as the BPRS, by the RSW who obtained information from the patient's family, place of employment, their agencies involved with the patient, as well as from the Summary Sheet obtained from the Camarillo State Hospital, filled out after the patient's release.

Design of Experiment

The design used is a balanced one in respect to race and sex, including the four plans of psychiatric management and the four treating psychiatrists. The validation was shown by the degree of agreement in the scores of the BPRS simultaneously and independently rated by two nontreating psychiatrists on a random subsample of patients.

A number of significant questions were tested in this project, among them the following:

A. What relationship exists between the BPRS and HVRS in respect to psychopathology scores?

B. What relationship exists between the changes in the psychopathology scores BPRS and HVRS on each of the following: (1) drug thioridazine versus placebo; (2) maximal versus minimal psychiatric care; (3) at different time intervals: admission to the clinic, during the clinical trial, from three to 12 weeks; at follow-up (average mean three months); (4) socialization, employment, recreational adjustment, and overall functioning; (5) contention in conjugal and lineal family; (6) male and female patients on admission and at follow-up?

C. What relationship exists between thioridazine and placebo and the following: (1) overall functioning of the patient; (2) contention in conjugal and lineal family?

Whenever we had a sufficient number of patients in our experimental sample, we used association tests: χ^2 was estimated. When $P < 0.05$, we reported the variable. We were compelled to use small samples because of situations beyond our control, such as the closing of the LASMHC due to state budget cut.

RESULTS

As previously indicated, our hospitalized patient population was treated for a short period of time: a mean average of 2.1 months at the Camarillo State Hospital, mainly with phenothiazines and milieu therapy. We also have indicated that our continuous communication with the patient and his family, from his admission to the hospital through his departure and release, made the significant difference between the number of patients who came for treatment and those who did not. A comparison between the general clinic and our own aftercare treatment of continuous communication presented a highly significant difference in our favor, in respect to patients arriving for treatment who remained for 12 weeks. What is important is that when continuous communication was used by the general clinic staff with their patients, the results were not significantly different.

We also discovered that ten patients came once and seven patients dropped out of the ECDEU project during 12 weeks of treatment; three patients relapsed and needed rehospitalization; and 40 patients stayed three to 12 weeks during the clinical trial. We were able to measure 39 patients who had remained nine to 15 weeks of the clinical trial and had a BPRS. At the end, we were able to follow up a sample that ranged around 40 patients who had had either a BPRS or an HVRS.

Although we used a balanced design, placing patients on maximal and minimal psychiatric care, a majority of patients, because of absences, did not follow the *maximal* program; thus, generally they became, by their own choice, patients who received *minimal psychiatric care*. Not only did this happen with the temporal involvement of care, but also with drugs versus placebo. The majority refused to take the amount of drug scheduled in the design, the result being an average mean taking 150 mg of thioridazine and 1.5 capsules of placebo. The reason given for not taking the capsules as prescribed was that they needed them only for sleep. Patients who were relapsing accepted more medication than the average mean. Our reports relative to the amount of drugs taken by the patients were as accurate as we could obtain by interviewing the family, the patient, and significant others. Therefore, in our calculations we could not make a comparison between maximal and minimal psychiatric care. Nor could an adequate comparison between drug and placebo be determined, since drugs taken were 150 mg. The chief observations made were that in every case they accepted the milieu of moral treatment and the quality of the relationships the ECDEU project offered in overcoming the obstructions of the "here and now."

Data about the patient population is noted in Table 3. There was a stratification of sex, a racial distribution—about two thirds (65%)

TABLE 1

Admissions to Los Angeles State Mental Hygiene Clinic (LASMHC) Early Clinical Drug Evaluation Unit (ECDEU) Project from Camarillo State Hospital

No. of Admissions	To	% of Show-Ups*	%–No. of Weeks Completed†	χ^2
		Admissions First Three Months		
180	LASMHC	39.4%	22.2%–12 weeks	* $\chi^2 = 13.49$ P < .001
38	ECDEU	73.7%	31.6%–12 weeks	† $\chi^2 = 1.041$ P < .05
		Admissions Second Three Months		
183	LASMHC	42.6%	31.1%–12 weeks	* $\chi^2 = 20.5$ P < .001
26	ECDEU	92.3%	69.2%–12 weeks	† $\chi^2 = 12.74$ P < .001
		Admissions Last Six Weeks		
170	LASMHC	68.8%	60% –12 weeks	
16	ECDEU	68.8%	56.2%–12 weeks	

* Statistically   † Not Significant

TABLE 2

Comparison of Total Psychopathology of the Brief Psychiatric Rating Scale (BPRS)

Changes from Admission to Clinic Project (ADC) Through Clinical Trial Follow-Up[*] [†]

	Number	Percentage
Better	14	35.9%
No Change	16	41.0%
Worse	9	23.1%
	N = 39	100%

[*] Follow-up (mean average, 3 months).
[†] Ratio of worse to better not significantly different.

TABLE 3

Population of Project in Percentages

Age in Years	%	Sex %	Race %	Social Class	%
20–24	27.5	Male 47.5	White 65.0	1	2.5
25–29	7.5	Female 52.5	Negro 27.5	2	2.5
30–34	22.5		Other 7.5	3	35.0
35–39	17.5	100.0		4	60.0
40–44	12.5			5	0.0
45–49	12.5		100.0		100.0
	100.0				

Mean Age = 33.4 years

Marital Status %	Male	Female	Months of Hosp. Stay	%[*]
Single	47.4	19.0	Under 1	17.5
Married	47.4	66.7	1–2	42.5
Divorced	5.3	9.5	2–3	17.5
Widowed	0.0	4.8	3–4	10.0
			4–5	7.5
	100.1	100.0	5–6	5.0
				100.0

[*] Mean Length Hosp. Stay = 2.1 months

were white, 27.5% Negro, and 7.5% a mixture of races. The social class that predominated was the lower-middle, with the middle-middle class following closely (Hollingshead and Redlich's Classification, Classes 3 and 4^{31}). There were no patients of the lowest socio-economic class (Hollingshead and Redlich's Class 5) among the clinic samples. The final data showed that the mean length of hospital stay was equal to 2.1 months; 42.5% stayed under two months, and 17.5% less than one month. On departure from the state hospital the patient had had large doses of phenothiazines administered, which would be slowly excreted within several weeks to several months.[32] DiMascio shows in this volume that when medication is withdrawn, such as the phenothiazines, regression to previous schizophrenic symptoms may occur in a few months.

The marital status of the patients was as follows: males had a large single population, and less than 50% were married; close to 70% of the females were married. Less than 20% of the females had remained single. Females admitted to the clinic were more significantly disturbed; after follow-up, they were more significantly improved than the males.

TABLE 4

Degree of Psychopathology at Different Time Intervals

		Mild	Moderate	Total
	Psychopathology at Admission to Clinic			
	Male	16	3	19
	Female	8	10	18
	Total	24	13	37

$$\chi^2 = 4.79, \text{d.f.} = 1, P < .05$$

	Very Mild	Mild	Moderate	Severe	Total
	Psychopathology at Follow-Up				
Male	5	9	4	1	19
Female	10	3	3	5	21
Total	15	12	7	6	40

$$\chi^2 = 7.39, \text{d.f.} = 3, .10 < P < .05$$

ASSESSMENT OF PSYCHOPATHOLOGY AND ITS RELATIONSHIP WITH DIFFERENT VARIABLES

A study was made concerning the relationship between the BPRS and the HVRS and their respective psychopathology scores. On admission of 60 patients to the ECDEU, it was discovered that a great significance existed between these different assessments. The

TABLE 5

Comparison of Ratings of Degree of Psychopathology Using the Brief Psychiatric Rating Scale (BPRS) and the Home Visit Rating Scale (HVRS)

BPRS	Very Mild	Mild	HVRS Moderate	Severe	Total
Very Mild	12	4	0	0	16
Mild	2	4	1	0	7
Moderate	1	4	4	1	10
Severe	0	0	2	1	3
Total	15	12	7	2	36

$$\chi^2 = 20.97, \text{d.f.} = 4, P < .001$$

For the purpose of the test, the moderate and severe categories had to be combined.

importance of this finding demonstrates the strong relationship present between these scales relative to psychopathology.

A further study was made measured in percentages between the relationship of degree of psychopathology that occurred at different time intervals, HVRS. On admission to the clinic, very mild and mild psychopathology scaled 65% with mild psychopathology 35%. During the clinic-trial period of three to 12 weeks, the very mild and mild psychopathology scaled 59%, the moderate 30%, and the severe about 10%.

On follow-up—mean average, three months—the very mild and mild psychopathology became 67%, the moderate 16%, and the severe increased slightly to 16%.

Table 6 also reveals the following findings: Although some patients improved during the clinical trial, some became worse, and on follow-up the same degree of psychopathology was sustained—that is, a number became milder and a number became more severe;

TABLE 6

Percent Comparison of Ratings of Psychopathology Using the Home Visit Rating Scale (HVRS)

Psychopathology	Admission to Clinic Project	During Trial*	Follow-Up (FU)†
Very Mild	8.1	20.5	35.1
Mild	56.8	38.5	32.4
Moderate	35.1	30.8	16.2
Severe	0.0	10.3	16.2
Total	100.0	100.1	99.9 .

* Three to twelve weeks.
† Follow-up (mean average, three months).

TABLE 7

Comparison of Psychopathology After Treatment Using the Home Visit Rating Scale (HVRS) from Admission to Clinic Project to Follow-Up*

	Better	No Change	Somewhat Worse	Much Worse	Total
Thioridazine	4	10	1	4	19
Placebo	5	7	4	2	18
Total	9	17	5	6	37†

No significant difference between Drug and Placebo

* Three months clinical trial plus mean average three-months follow-up.
† 3, unknown ADC.

generally, however, the patients were able to sustain their degree of psychopathology. Only 10% became severe during the clinical trial, and 16% during the follow-up.

A comparison was made after treatment with drug (thioridazine) or placebo at two time intervals: on admission to the clinic, and at follow-up. Using the HVRS as an assessment, we found no significant difference between drug and placebo. When a comparison was made of the therapeutic response to drug and placebo between the contention in the family at follow-up and disturbance in function (socialization, employment, recreational adjustment), no significant difference was discovered between drug and placebo; this held throughout our study. We were most cautious in our search for significant differences, since we were biased in favor of the drug.

TABLE 8

Relationship of Therapeutic Response to Drug and Placebo

	Very Mild	Mild	Moderate	Severe	Total
Contention in the Family at Follow-Up					
Drug					
(Thioridazine)	7	7	1	1	16
Placebo	3	4	6	0	13
Total	10	11	7	1	29
Disturbance in Function at Follow-Up					
Drug					
(Thioridazine)	7	11	0	3	21
Placebo	3	13	3	0	19
Total	10	24	3	3	40

No significant difference between Drug and Placebo

TABLE 9

Comparison of Total Psychopathology of the Brief Psychiatric Rating Scale (BPRS)

Changes from Admission to Clinic Project (ADC) Through Clinical Trial* (9–15 weeks) †

	Number	Percentage
Better	8	32%
No Change	16	64%
Worse	1	4.0%
	N = 25	100.0%

Changes from Admission to Clinic Project (ADC) Through Clinical Trial to Follow-Up‡ §

	Number	Percentage
Better	14	35.9%
No Change	16	41.0%
Worse	9	23.1%
	N = 39	100.0%

* Clinical trial—mean average, 13 weeks.
† Significantly better $P < .05$.
‡ Follow-up—mean average, 3 months.
§ Ratio of worse to better not significantly different.

We did a comparison (Table 9) of the total psychopathology of the BPRS, the changes being studied from admission to the clinic through the clinical trial period of nine to 15 weeks. (See first part of Table 9.) The comparison showed 64% unchanged, 32% better, and 4% worse.

The changes observed from clinic admission through the period of the clinical trial and extending to the follow-up showed the following: Those who were better reached a level of 35.9%; 41% remained unchanged, and 23.1% became worse. Thus, approximately 77% of the patients either improved or did not change. After an average of six months of treatment and follow-up, the patients' improvement symptoms were sustained without regressing toward severity (see last part of Table 9).

TABLE 10

Comparison of Brief Psychiatric Rating Scale (BPRS) Items with Similar Scores at Admission to Clinic Project & During Clinical Trial (9–15 Weeks)

1. SOMATIC CONCERN
2. ANXIETY
3. EMOTIONAL WITHDRAWAL
4. CONCEPTUAL DISORGANIZATION
5. GUILT FEELINGS
6. TENSION
7. MANNERISMS AND POSTURING
8. GRANDIOSITY
9. DEPRESSION
10. HOSTILITY
11. SUSPICIOUSNESS
12. HALLUCINATORY BEHAVIOR
13. MOTOR RETARDATION
14. UNCOOPERATIVENESS
15. UNUSUAL THOUGHT CONTENT
16. BLUNTED AFFECT
17. INAPPROPRIATE AFFECT
18. EXCITEMENT
19. DISORIENTATION
20. IMPAIRED MEMORY
21. IMPAIRED JUDGMENT AND PLANNING
22. PSYCHONEUROTIC SYMPTOMS
23. THINKING DISTURBANCE
24. INTERPERSONAL DISTURBANCE
25. WITHDRAWAL RETARDATION
26. TENSION-EXCITEMENT
27. DEPRESSIVE DISTURBANCE
28. INAPPROPRIATE AFFECT
29. TOTAL PSYCHIATRIC PATHOLOGY*
30. SPECIFIC ITEMS (1–18)†
31. GENERAL ITEMS (23–28)‡
32. UNSCORED ITEMS (19–22)

* $\chi^2 = 9.0327$, d.f. $= 2$, P $< .05$.
† $\chi^2 = 6.0268$, d.f. $= 2$, P $< .05$.
‡ $\chi^2 = 6.4352$, d.f. $= 2$, P $< .05$.

A comparison made of the BPRS item scores measured on admission to the clinic and on nine to 15 weeks determined that specific BPRS items 1–18, and the general mean score of items 23–28, were highly significant: the measurement of the patients' BPRS score items remained unchanged. This documented the evidence to show the patient's BPRS scores remained stable during the trial period.

Our experiment made a study of the relationship of psychopathology to the disturbance of patients' function in their community roles and contention within the conjugal and lineal families. Using the HVRS, we divided the above into the following categories, and ascertained these results:

TABLE 11

Relation of Psychopathology as Shown by Home Visit Rating Scale (HVRS) to Disturbance of Function and to Contention in Family at Time of Follow-Up

	Very Mild	Mild	Moderate or Severe	Total
Disturbance in Socialization				
Very Mild	13	7	2	22
Mild	2	5	3	10
Moderate or Severe	0	0	8	8
Total	15	12	13	40

$$\chi^2 = 25.25, \text{d.f.} = 4, \text{P} < .001$$

	Very Mild	Mild	Moderate or Severe	Total
Employment				
Very Mild	8	3	1	12
Mild	7	4	5	16
Moderate or Severe	0	5	7	12
Total	15	12	13	40

$$\chi^2 = 12.79, \text{d.f.} = 4, \text{P} < .05$$

1. *Disturbance in Socialization.* There was a significant relationship between the disturbance of psychopathology and socialization, with most of the patients being able to reach a high level of socialization whether moderately or severely disturbed. The largest number of patients had very mild to mild disturbances; they made good adaptation to social situations.

2. *Employment* (*Education, Housewives*). (See Table 11.) There was a significant relationship between degree of psychopathology and employment. Those patients who were employed or continuing their education or managing households tended to show less disturbance. With the number of our severely disturbed cases being extremely small, a significant majority would appear to have achieved a good adaptation to their employment or educational environment within the community.

TABLE 12

Relation of Psychopathology as Shown by Home Visit Rating Scale (HVRS) to Disturbance of Function and to Contention in Family at Time of Follow-Up

	Very Mild	Mild	Moderate or Severe	Total
Recreational Adjustment				
None	5	1	2	8
Very Mild	6	8	2	16
Mild	4	2	1	7
Moderate or Severe	0	1	8	9
Total	15	12	13	40

$$\chi^2 = 21.08, \text{d.f.} = 6, P < .01$$

	Very Mild	Mild	Moderate or Severe	Total
*Contention in Family**				
Very Mild	8	1	0	9
Mild	3	1	5	9
Moderate or Severe	1	6	4	11
Total	12	8	9	29†

* Trend showing a relationship in percentage of degree of psychopathology and contention in family. χ^2 not valid because of small numbers.

† This item was not applicable for the remaining 11 patients.

3. *Recreational Adjustment.* In a similar manner, the patient's recreational adjustment was dependent on the degree of psychopathology. The milder the degree of psychopathology, the more likely the patient was to have an excellent recreational adjustment. The majority of our patient population made a significantly good adaptation to recreational adjustment.

4. *Contention in the Family* (Conjugal and Lineal). (See Table 12.) Better family adjustment was evidenced by the majority of patients whose psychopathology was milder. However, since we had

too small a sampling, χ^2 could not be calculated as an association test. From so small a sampling we were nevertheless able to establish a reasonable observation that the family relationship had a direct bearing on the degree of the patient's psychopathology. A larger number of patients were needed to obtain a statistically significant result.

TABLE 13

Relation of Psychopathology as Shown by Home Visit Rating Scale (HVRS) to Disturbance of Function and to Contention in Family at Time of Follow-Up

	Very Mild	Mild	Moderate or Severe	Total
Disturbance in Function				
None	8	2	0	10
Mild	7	8	4	19
Moderate or Severe	0	2	9	11
Total	15	12	13	40

$$\chi^2 = 22.97, \text{d.f.} = 4, P < .001$$

5. *Disturbance in Function.* If all the functions in the community, such as socialization, employment, recreational adjustment, and contention in family were added and scored together, we would come to the conclusion that an extremely significant relationship existed between the degree of psychopathology and disturbance in function. (See Table 13.) In brief, the majority of our patients, having very mild, mild, or moderate disturbances, were able to function extremely well in the community, and their psychopathology did not prevent them from making a good adaptation on these levels. Most patients held the therapeutic gains made at the state hospital and were sustained by their treatment at the ECDEU of the LASMHC.

DISCUSSION

We tested out a number of hypotheses involving the early schizophrenic who had a first hospital admission. The main treatment at the State of California Camarillo State Hospital was psychopharmacotherapy. The schizophrenic's nonpharmacologic treatments included the hospital milieu, relationship with the general staff, and, in a few cases, group psychotherapy. We then followed the patient, after release, to an outpatient aftercare center in the Los Angeles area near his community. At the facility where the patient was treated, the LASMHC and ECDEU research team was in residence. Here treatment varied in complexity in the degree of temporal involvement of the doctor-patient relationship, the degree of the treatment milieu, the social therapy, including family therapy, and the use of drugs or placebo in a double-blind design experiment.

The results discussed above show that the patient who had continuous communication with our research unit from early admission, through Camarillo State Hospital, to his reintegration into the community cooperated much more frequently than the general patient who came to the aftercare clinic. When the general aftercare clinic followed our unit's methods and procedures to alleviate the fragmentation of the patient, the clinic's "no-shows" were of a similar percentage to our project's, 20% to 25%. (See Table 1.)

As indicated in Table 3, socio-economic classes were mainly from the lower-middle, with a small but significant group from the middle-middle class. There is a possibility that our unit's "no-show" group could have come chiefly from the lowest socio-economic level. This assumption can be in part related, of course, to the general behavioral patterns of the lowest socio-economic level, who do not conform to good attendance at psychiatric facilities. The problem of treating the disadvantaged at a clinic facility is the patient's refusal to come for treatment. Another observation is that the majority of patients evinced a general resistance toward following any set research design. This is not unusual. The resistance was greatest in two areas: first, in accepting any maximal psychiatric care requiring large involvements of time or frequency of visits; second, refusal to take prescribed doses of thioridazine and placebo. Instead of taking three to four capsules per day, which is an average dose for a psychotic, patients averaged about 1.5 capsules (150 mg) of drug and 1.5 capsules of placebo.

The reasons for this general resistance by the patients is evidenced by this chapter's statistical tables. When the patient had mild psychopathology to moderate disturbance, his general movement was toward reintegrating himself quickly into the community and his family. From our interviews with such patients, our distinct impression was that their situation seemed favorable to them and therefore they felt little need of any treatment—just enough medication to act as a sleeping pill. Other reasons they did not come to the clinic were that it interfered with their working, transportation was expensive, the problem of getting off from work or school insurmountable and embarrassing, and getting a sitter for the children expensive. The cost to the patient who was functioning was too high.

The ECDEU cases treated in the present experiment, when leaving Camarillo State Hospital and released by the hospital physician, were directed toward our clinic by our social worker. Both physician and social worker were optimistic that the patient could get along in the community with aftercare alone, thus encouraging the patient clinically toward further improvement. Phenothiazines, previously taken in relatively large doses, could help temporarily to sustain the patient in the community, until complete withdrawal was effected. In addition, hospital treatments could aid toward bolstering a patient for a length of time before possible relapse would occur. (Caffey, et al; May, et al.) Since the remission in schizophrenia is less than 40%, rehospitalization about 60%, and relapse after discharge high, we may reasonably speculate that other factors than previous hospital treatment operated during six months' aftercare treatment.

Our results seem impressive with this subtype of patient. Engelhardt, et al, have rated hospital-prone schizophrenic patients and their clinical course during phenothiazine treatment. Our observations, which their research confirmed in another area of the nation, indicate there are hypothetical subtypes of schizophrenic patients whose therapeutic responses could be encouraged by drugs or moral treatment alone or combined. We had speculated that we had preselected for treatment from the general population of the Camarillo State Hospital a cohort of therapeutically responsive, early, first-admission schizophrenic patients. A study of our criteria will show how we may have selected patients who have favorable prognoses. It is therefore not surprising that this cohort synchronized and reinforced our form of moral treatment. Another deduction follows that many previously hospitalized patients could have been treated in the community with modified moral treatment—that is, minimal psychotherapeutic management, minimal drug therapy, and minimal social therapy.

We feel it is most necessary that our experiment be replicated by a much larger number of patients with better controls and a follow-up of two years of treated patients. Using the same criteria of selection for a similar group of early, first-admission schizophrenics, we would like them to be followed without any treatment for comparison to the above-treated patients.

As we have pointed out, LAMHC had a large dropout rate for aftercare of about 75%. The ECDEU project in the clinic had a dropout rate that varied from 25% and increased on follow-up. Because there is a general reluctance on the part of the patients to follow our intensive care design, we must devise new techniques that will create a tighter and more workable design. The patients' reluctance to follow our design and the dropouts were mainly due to the large interference that treatment produces in their way of life; their main purpose is to reintegrate themselves into their community and family environment.

In order to increase our ECDEU subjects and decrease the dropout rate we must follow a new strategy. The reluctance of the patients to accept intensive care can be resolved. In order to keep the design of our experiment as it was, we can perform our investigation by having half the patients' psychiatric care at home and half at the clinic. Those at the clinic may have minimal care and those being treated at home maximal treatment. The drug that should be used in maximal or minimal care should be an intramuscular injection of fluphenazine decanoate or placebo in order to avoid patients' choices of dosages. Intensive individual psychotherapy can be given at home with family therapy, in addition to intramuscular fluphenazine decanoate.[16-18] In this fashion the comparison between patients who receive intensive versus minimal care then can be carried out, and the dropout rate be markedly reduced.

In closing: Though this research project is but one additional piece of evidence in a series, it indicates that our form of moral treatment is a significant factor in helping patients to rid themselves of their dehumanization.

Many of our past and present therapies—somatic, psychotherapeutic, administrative, and hospital treatment—have frequently fragmented the person in need of help. The mental health center is a new organizational approach containing many excellent intentions and many uncertain results. Its success might depend to a considerable extent on its ability to humanize the patient.

Conclusions and Summary

1. We investigated a subtype of early acute schizophrenic patients who had one hospital admission and a number of other criteria

enumerated below. This group had a mean of 2.1 months of treatment at Camarillo State Hospital prior to release to our ECDEU project at the LASMHC.

2. Consistent attendance at the clinic was related to making early rapport and contact with the family and patient early in their hospitalization and continuing this open-end approach throughout the project.

3. Most patients belonged to the middle-middle and lower-middle class, and chose their own treatment, strongly resisting certain portions of our research plan. They generally chose concise minimal psychiatric management and relatively small doses of psychoactive drugs or placebo. Only three were rehospitalized.

4. The Brief Psychiatric Rating Scale (BPRS) and the Home Visit Rating Scale (HVRS) gave highly significant similar results in respect to psychopathology of our cohort of patients, and could be used interchangeably.

5. During the clinical trial and at follow-up there was generally little change in psychopathology scores—ie, the results showed that patients remained 67% mildly ill, 16% moderately ill, and 16% severely ill after treatment and follow-up (average mean, six months).

6. There were no significant differences between psychoactive drug and placebo in the double-blind study as measured by the total overall functioning of the patient in the community and in respect to contention in the family.

7. The degree of psychopathology was directly proportional, and statistically significant, to disturbance in socialization, employment, recreational adjustment, and contention in family. This was similar when total overall functioning of the patient was compared to degree of psychopathology.

8. Above all, the project revealed that after an initial brief hospitalization our subtype of early acute schizophrenic could be maintained in the community with minimal psychiatric management and no psychoactive drugs, and that their psychopathology remained generally unchanged after six months' follow-up, with rare rehospitalization.

REFERENCES

1. *Community Mental Health Center: Analysis of Existing Models,* Washington, D.C.: Joint Information Service of American Psychiatric Association and National Association for Mental Health, 1964, p. 11.
2. Freeman, H. E., and Simmons, O. C.: *The Mental Patient Comes Home,* New York: John Wiley & Sons, 1963.
3. Bockhoven, J. S.: *Moral Treatment in American Psychiatry,* New York: Springer Publishing Company, 1963.
4. Rees, T. P.: Back to Moral Treatment and Community Care, *J. Ment. Sci.,* vol. 103, 43:303–313, April, 1957.
5. Rothman, T.: Moral Treatment and Psychopharmacology in Day Treatment Center; Study Group Proceedings, A.C.N.P., Washington, D.C.: *Psychopharmacol. Serv. Ctr. Bull.,* 1965.
6. Kraepelin, E.: *One Hundred Years of Psychiatry* (trans. by W. Baskin from 1917 edition), Berlin: Springer Verlag; New York: 1962, p. 155.
7. Hodern, A., and Hamilton, M.: Drugs and Moral Treatment, *Brit. J. Psych.,* 109:500–509, 1963.
8. Joint Commission on Mental Illness and Health: Research Resources in Mental Health, *Action for Mental Health: Final Report of General Commission on Mental Illness and Health,* New York: Basic Books, 1961, pp. 193–224.
9. Katz, M., and Cole, J. O.: Phenomenological Approach to Classification of Schizophrenic Disorders, *Dis. Nerv. Syst.,* 24 (No. 3), 1963.
10. Glasscote, et al: *Community Health Center: Interim Appraisal,* Washington, D.C.: Joint Information Service of American Psychiatric Association and National Association for Mental Health, 1969, pp. 31–32.
11. Glasscote, et al: *Partial Hospitalization for the Mentally Ill: Study of Programs and Problems,* Washington, D.C.: Joint Information Service of American Psychiatric Association and National Association for Mental Health, 1969.
12. Greenblatt, M., et al: *Mental Patients in Transition:* Springfield, Ill., Charles C. Thomas, 1965.
13. Epps, R. L., Barnes, R. H., and McPartland, T. S.: *A Community Concern:* Springfield, Ill., Charles C. Thomas, 1965.
14. Zusman, J.: "Some Explanations of Changing Appearance of Psychotic Patients: Antecedents of Social Breakdown Syndrome," in Gruenberg, E. M. (ed.): *Evaluating Effectiveness of Community Health Services,* New York: Milbank Memorial Fund, 1966, pp. 363–391.
15. Grad, J., and Sainsbury, P.: "Evaluation of a Community Care Service," in *Trends in Mental Health,* New York: Macmillan, 1963, pp. 177–220.
16. Pasamanick, B., and Scapitta, A.: Problems in Home Care for Schizophrenia, *Arch. Gen. Psychiat.,* 10:143–154, 1964.
17. Friedman, T., Rolfe, P., and Perry, S. P.: Home Treatment of Schizophrenia, *Admin. J. Psych.,* 1960.
18. Friedman, T., and Weiner, L.: "Psychiatric Home Services," in *Current Psychiatric Therapies,* vol. 5, New York: Grune & Stratton, 1965, pp. 186–201.
19. Dondis, E. H.: "Methods for Evaluating Day Treatment Centers," in *Transitional Psychiatric Settings,* San Diego: San Diego Day Treatment Center Foundation, 1962.

20. McMillan, T. M., and Dondis, E. H.: Treatment and Research at Day Treatment Center, *Dis. Nerv. Syst.*, 24:360–364, 1963.
21. Kris, E. B.: Drug Therapy in a Day Care Facility for Relapse Control; Study Group Proceedings, A.C.N.P., *Psychopharmacol. Serv. Ctr. Bull.*, 1965.
22. Rothman, T.: Concise Minimal Psychotherapy Combined with Drugs: Study Group Proceedings, Washington, D.C.: *Bull.* A.C.N.P., 1964.
23. Hamilton, M., et al: A Controlled Trial on the Value of Prochlorperazine, Trifluoperazine and Intensive Group Treatment, *Brit. J. Psychiat.*, 109:510–522, 1963.
24. Tourney, G.: History of Therapeutic Fashion in Psychiatry, 1800–1965, *Amer. J. Psychiat.*, 124, 1967.
25. Greenblatt, M., et al: *Drugs and Social Therapy in Chronic Schizophrenia*, Springfield, Ill.: Charles C. Thomas, 1965.
26. Engelhardt, D. M., et al: Prevention of Psychiatric Hospitalization with Use of Psychopharmacological Agents, *JAMA*, 173:147–149, 1960.
27. Engelhardt, D. M., et al: Phenothiazines in Prevention of Psychiatric Hospitalization: II. Duration of Treatment Exposure, *JAMA*, 186:981–983, 1963.
28. Engelhardt, D. M., et al: Phenothiazines in Prevention of Psychiatric Hospitalization: III. Prevention or Delay of Hospitalization, *Arch. Gen. Psychiat.*, 11:162–169, 1964.
29. Engelhardt, D. M., et al: Phenothiazines in Prevention of Psychiatric Hospitalization: IV. Delay or Prevention of Hospitalization: Reevaluation, *Arch. Gen. Psychiat.*, 16:98–102, 1967.
30. Whittington, H. C.: *Psychiatry in the American Community*, New York: International University Press, Inc., 1966, pp. 293–304.
31. Hollingshead, A. B., and Redlich, F. C.: *Social Class and Mental Illness: Community Study*, New York: John Wiley & Sons, 1958.
32. Caffey, E. M., Jr., et al: Discontinuation or Reduction of Chemotherapy in Chronic Schizophrenics, *J. Chronic Dis.*, 17:347, 1964.

8

*High Dose Chlorpromazine Therapy in Chronic Schizophrenia**

by ROBERT F. PRIEN

and JONATHAN O. COLE

Prien and Cole, in a collaborative study involving 838 chronic schizo-phrenics in seven public mental hospitals, compared a high-dose chlorpro-mazine regimen (2,000 mg/day) with chlorpromazine 300 mg/day, a placebo, and routine hospital treatment. Treatment followed a double-blind procedure for 24 weeks with patients under 40 years of age and hospitalized less than ten years. It was found that high dose was signifi-cantly more effective than low dose, placebo, or routine treatment. Changes included a wide range of schizophrenic symptoms, especially in psychosocial adequacies and community adjustment potential—two areas of social adjustment known to be related to release from the mental hospital.

* Published in the Archives of General Psychiatry, Vol. 18, April 1968, and re-printed with permission. This investigation was supported by Public Health Service grants MH–10292, MH–11384, MH–10496, MH–10989, MH–11046, MH–11047, and MH–10332, from the National Institute of Mental Health, and Public Health Service contract SA–43–ph–3064. Data was contributed by the following individuals and their staff from the seven participating hospitals: Edwin M. Davidson, M.D., and Melvin M. Kayce, M.D., Boston State Hospital; Thomas A. Smith, M.D., Broughton State Hospital; Myron G. Sandifer, M.D., and William J. Buffaloe, M.D., Dorothea Dix State Hospital; William J. Kernohan, M.D., and Winston T. Wilson, Ph.D., Kentucky State Hospital; Herman C. Denber, M.D., and Edwin Meshel, M.D., Man-hattan State Hospital; Robert R. Knowles, M.D., B.S., D.P.M., and Cecil G. Baker, M.D., St. Louis State Hospital; Martin Gross, M.D., and Arthur Mandel, M.D., Springfield State Hospital.

Roland R. Bonato, Ph.D., Frances H. Fleming, M.N., and Naomi F. Hartwick of the Biometric Laboratory, George Washington University, and Solomon C. Goldberg, Ph.D., and Gerald E. Hogarty, M.S.W., Psychopharmacology Research Branch, Na-tional Institute of Mental Health, assisted in this study.

This chapter gives us therapeutic guidance and hope for patients younger than 40, anticipating that these particularly might additionally benefit from community care and become reintegrated members. Following a high-dosage schedule and release from the mental hospital facility, the special type of treatment of this subgroup of schizophrenics needs to be further investigated. The problem of reintegrating such patients into the community, including the amount of chlorpromazine needed in this long-term treatment and the potential occupational and family functioning, requires special study.

This Prien-Cole investigation should lead to worthwhile research.

This study on the efficacy of high dose chlorpromazine (Thorazine) treatment in chronic schizophrenia was developed under the National Institute of Mental Health (NIMH) psychopharmacology program during 1964, and was initiated in seven collaborating public mental hospitals early in 1965. The hospitals participating in this study included Boston State Hospital, Boston; Broughton State Hospital, Morganton, NC; Dorothea Dix State Hospital, Raleigh, NC; Kentucky State Hospital, Danville, Ky; Manhattan State Hospital, New York; St. Louis State Hospital, St. Louis; and Springfield State Hospital, Sykesville, Md. These hospitals were selected to represent the entire urban-rural continuum. Three of these hospitals admitted patients exclusively from large urban centers; two served areas that included both urban and rural communities, and two served areas that were almost exclusively rural.

BACKGROUND

During the past 13 years a large number of studies have been published on the use of chlorpromazine (Thorazine) with chronic schizophrenic patients. Although a majority of these studies indicated that chlorpromazine is effective in the treatment of chronic schizophrenia, there is considerable confusion and contradiction regarding matters of dosage, particularly the value of high dose schedules. Some investigators advocate the use of high doses; others contend that low doses are just as effective and less dangerous.[1-9] A review of the literature reveals a surprising paucity of controlled studies comparing high and low doses in the chronic schizophrenic patient. Several small studies in the mid-1950s compared different dose levels of chlorpromazine, but none of these studies used doses exceeding 600 mg/day. Only one comparative study reported in the literature used relatively high doses of chlorpromazine. Schiele[9] compared a high dose regimen of 1,400 to 3,000 mg with a low dose regimen of 300 to 1,400 mg in 38 male chronic schizophrenics. Although the results suggested that the high dose treatment was more effective, the authors acknowledged that methodological considerations made any interpretation of results tenuous.

There is also disagreement among investigators regarding optimum duration of treatment. Several investigators stress the importance of administering high doses to chronic patients for several months, [3, 8, 10] believing that many authors have drawn premature conclusions from experience with high dose therapy administered for too short a period of time.

Thus, after more than a decade of research on chlorpromazine, the question of high dose efficacy remains essentially unanswered. It is a question that has important therapeutic implications. In most public mental hospitals the majority of chronic schizophrenics are treated with low doses of phenothiazines. A presumed but unknown proportion have never received phenothiazine therapy at a very high dosage for a long period of time. The principal aim of this study was to determine whether these chronic schizophrenics would show major improvement if high doses were administered in a carefully supervised manner over a prolonged period of time.

RESEARCH QUESTIONS

This study was designed to respond to the following questions:

1. Is a high dose of 2,000 mg of chlorpromazine, administered over a prolonged period of time, more effective than a low dose of 300 mg typically used in the treatment of chronic schizophrenia?

2. Is high dose chlorpromazine more advantageous than treatment routinely administered to the chronic schizophrenic in the public mental hospital?

3. Are the two dose levels of chlorpromazine and the routine hospital treatment more effective than an inert placebo?

4. Do the treatments operate differentially on specific schizophrenic symptoms? For example, is high dose more effective than low dose in reducing delusional thinking?

5. Is there a type of patient who responds to one treatment and not to another?

6. What proportion of chronic patients shows an exacerbation of symptoms following withdrawal of regular medication and initiation of placebo?

7. Are there differences between treatments in the nature and/or frequency of side effects?

PROCEDURE

Approximately 120 chronic schizophrenics, stratified by sex, were selected at each of the seven hospitals by the following criteria:

1. A primary diagnosis of schizophrenia
2. Age between 19 and 55
3. Continuous hospitalization of at least two years. (Continuous hospitalization was defined as no more than eight weeks out of the hospital at any one time during the current stay.)
4. No evidence of the following clinical disorders:
    a. Organic brain disease, including lobotomy
    b. Mental deficiency (intelligence quotient below 70)
    c. Medical conditions contraindicating use of high doses.

In addition, patients were required to show symptoms, signs, or behavior in one or more of the following categories: perceptual disturbance, delusional thinking, thinking and speech disorganization, withdrawal, mannerisms and posturing, and lack of social competence.

Patients meeting these selection criteria were randomly assigned to four treatment groups: (1) high dose—2,000 mg of chlorpromazine per day; (2) low dose—300 mg of chlorpromazine per day; (3) placebo; and (4) routine—conventional hospital treatment. The last group consisted of patients who received whatever medication or dose the hospital chose to administer. The total number of patients in each treatment group was as follows: high dose, 208; low dose, 208; placebo, 212; and routine treatment, 210.

All patients were rated on psychiatric, nursing, and social work scales prior to entry into the study. Patients were then observed on their routine hospital medication for eight weeks, during which time physical and ophthalmologic examinations were performed. At the end of the eight-week baseline period, ratings were repeated and patients who had been assigned to high, low, and placebo groups were shifted to study medication. The routine-treatment group continued to receive hospital-determined medication. The high dose group received liquid concentrate chlorpromazine in gradually increasing dosage according to a predetermined schedule, reaching the maximum level of 2,000 mg after 45 days. Patients were maintained at that level for the remainder of a 24-week period. Permanent dose reduction to 1,500 mg was permitted to control for side effects. The low dose and placebo groups also received liquid concentrate, on a double-blind basis, for a 24-week period.

Assessment of Clinical Change

Clinical change was assessed in three ways. First, the doctor made overall clinical judgments of severity of illness and degree of improvement. Second, specific psychopathology was rated by the doctors on the basis of interviews, and by nurses on the basis of ward behavior. Third, readiness for discharge was evaluated by social workers from interviews and observations of ward behavior. The assessment instruments used by the doctors, nurses, and social workers are described below:

The Discharge Readiness Inventory (DRI), developed by Hogarty et al,[11] to evaluate release potential in the chronic schizophrenic patient was completed by the social worker twice for each patient, once prior to treatment and once at the conclusion of treatment. The DRI consists of 62 items, which have been factor-analyzed to form four independent subscales. Factor 1, Psychosocial Adequacy, measures the level of patient adjustment within the hospital. Factor 2, Belligerence, measures the degree of hostility and obstreperous behavior. Factor 3, Community Adjustment Potential, measures the patient's capacity for adjustment in the community. Factor 4, Manifest Psychopathology, measures the extent to which the patient's behavior is disrupted by hallucinations and delusions.

A validation study on the DRI was conducted prior to the collaborative study to determine whether the DRI actually discriminated between the discharge-ready and non-ready patient. At five of the collaborating hospitals, a total of 206 discharge-ready patients were evaluated on the DRI. These patients were chronic schizophrenics who had been referred to social service for discharge and had been judged discharge-ready by three independent judges: the referring psychiatrist, the social worker accepting the referral, and the research social worker. The discharge-ready patients were compared with chronic schizophrenics meeting collaborative study criteria. All four DRI factors significantly discriminated between the two groups of patients. Among the four DRI factors, Community

Adjustment Potential and Psychosocial Adequacy discriminated best between the ready and non-ready patients. The discharge-ready patient was best characterized by high positive scores on these two factors. Complete results from this validation study are presented elsewhere.[12] What is important in this regard is that all four DRI factors, particularly Community Adjustment Potential and Psychosocial Adequacy, proved to be valid measures of discharge readiness.

Inpatient Multidimensional Psychiatric Scale (IMPS). This was developed by Lorr, et al.[13] It consists of 81 symptom descriptions completed by the psychiatrist or clinical psychologist on the basis of a one-hour interview. The scale has been factor-analyzed to form ten independent subscales:

1. Excitement
2. Hostile–Belligerence
3. Paranoid Projection
4. Grandiose Expansiveness
5. Perceptual Distortions
6. Anxious Intropunitiveness
7. Retardation and Apathy
8. Disorientation
9. Motor Disturbances
10. Conceptual Disorganization

Each patient was evaluated on the IMPS prior to treatment and at eight-week intervals during treatment.

Nurse's Observation Scale for Inpatient Evaluation (NOSIE). Developed by Honigfeld, et al,[14] this scale consists of 80 items for evaluating the patient's behavior on the ward. The NOSIE has been factor-analyzed to form seven independent subscales:

1. Social Competence
2. Social Interest
3. Cooperation
4. Personal Neatness
5. Irritability
6. Manifest Psychosis
7. Paranoid Depression

The NOSIE was completed by the research nurse prior to treatment and at eight-week intervals during treatment.

Global Assessments. Two global scales were completed by the doctor at the conclusion of the IMPS interview:

A. Global Improvement Scale: "Compared to his condition at the start of treatment, how much has the patient changed?"—(1) very much improved; (2) much improved; (3) slightly improved; (4) no change; (5) minimally worse; (6) much worse; or (7) very much worse.

B. Global Severity of Illness Scale: "Considering your total clinical experience, how mentally ill is the patient at this time?"—(1) normal, not ill at all; (2) borderline mentally ill; (3) mildly ill; (4) moderately ill; (5) markedly ill; (6) severely ill; or (7) among the most extremely ill patients.

In addition to the DRI, IMPS, NOSIE, and global scales, a 40-item side-effect checklist was completed by the research physician and the research nurse. This checklist was completed prior to treatment and at two-week intervals during treatment. Side effects were rated slight, moderate, or severe in intensity. Each patient was also examined by an ophthalmologist prior to treatment, after 12 weeks of treatment, and at the conclusion of treatment.

Method of Analysis of Clinical Data

To avoid excessive length and complexity, this paper will deal only with comparisons involving the high dose group—ie, high dose versus low dose, high dose versus routine treatment, and high dose versus placebo. A subsequent paper will deal with comparisons among the other treatment groups—eg, low dose versus placebo.

Each patient was evaluated on 23 criterion measures: ten IMPS factors, seven NOSIE factors, four DRI factors, and two global scales. Except for the Global Improvement Scale, criterion measures were analyzed by analysis of covariance computed from a factorial design involving four treatment groups, two sexes, two age groups (under 40, over 40), and two levels of current hospitalization (under ten years, over ten years). The covariates were pretreatment scores, and the variates were scores obtained when the patient left the study. Both early terminators and patients who completed the full 24 weeks of treatment were included in the analysis. Each early terminator was evaluated at the time he was dropped from the study, and this score was used as the patient's variate measure in the analysis.

The covariance analyses showed either a significant drug main effect or significant drug interaction on all criterion measures. On the basis of these analyses, three additional covariance analyses were computed for each criterion measure. Each analysis was based on two treatments, two sexes, the two age levels, and the two lengths of hospitalization. The first analysis compared high dose and low dose, the second compared high dose and routine treatment, and the third compared high dose and placebo. When an analysis showed a significant drug interaction, a multiple range test[15] was employed to determine the significance of differences in the individual comparisons involved in the interaction. The 5% level of statistical significance was used in all analyses reported in this paper.

On each criterion measure, two-tailed *t*-tests for correlated samples were used to determine significance of change from pretreatment to posttreatment. Analyses were performed for each treatment group at each level of age and hospitalization.

RESULTS

Characteristics of the Sample at Start of Study

A description of study patients is presented in Table 1. The mean age of patients was 41.6 years, 61% being over 40 years of age. Total hospitalization ranged from two to 34 years, with a mean of 14.5 years. The mean duration of current hospitalization was 13.1 years; 57% of the patients had been hospitalized over ten years during the current stay.

The analysis of the social characteristics of the sample revealed that 84% of the men and 58% of the women had never been married. Twenty percent of the men and 40% of the women had never been employed; an additional 49% of the men and 19% of the women had worked only at unskilled jobs. Educational achievement was relatively poor—only 17% of the men and 28% of the women had completed high school.

Pretreatment symptomatology was analyzed by age and length of current hospitalization. The results showed that patients hospitalized less than ten years were markedly different from patients hospitalized over ten years. The less hospitalized patients showed significantly more florid schizophrenic symptomatology (conceptual, delusional, and perceptual disturbance), social competence, and social interest than the patients hospitalized over ten years. The latter group of patients were for the most part relatively inactive, showed severe social withdrawal, and exhibited little affect either in the form of excitement or depression.

TABLE 1

Background Characteristics of Study Patients

Characteristics		Male	Female	Total
Age at admission	Mean	40.8	42.4	41.6
to project	SD	9.0	7.7	8.4
	% over 39	58	66	62
Age at first	Mean	23.5	25.0	24.2
hospitalization	SD	5.9	6.8	6.4
Years current	Mean	13.3	13.0	13.1
hospitalization	SD	8.5	8.7	8.6
	% over 10	56	54	55
Years total	Mean	14.6	14.4	14.5
hospitalization	SD	8.1	8.1	8.1
	% over 10	63	63	63
	% over 20	26	26	26
Race	% White	89	90	89
Marital status	% married—now			
	or ever	16	42	28
Education	% attending			
	high school	43	54	48
	% completing			
	high school	17	28	22
Work history	% never employed	20	40	29
	% employed only			
	in unskilled jobs	49	19	35

Global Improvement Scale

Marked improvement occurred in 10% of the high dose group, 6% of the low dose group, 3% of the placebo group, and 3% of the routine treatment group. (For convenience, a patient rated "much improved" or "very much improved" on the Global Scale is referred to as markedly improved.) An additional 17% of the high dose group, 12% of the low dose group, 8% of the placebo group, and 14% of the routine treatment group were found to be slightly improved.

Table 2 presents global ratings by treatment group, age, and length of hospitalizations. The major results from Table 2 are summarized as follows:

Younger, Less Hospitalized Patients (Under 40, Hospitalized Under Ten Years).

The high dose treatment proved more effective than each of the

TABLE 2

Change in Global Psychiatric State by Treatment Group, Age, and Length of Current Hospitalization*

Age in Years	Years Currently in Hospital	Treatment Group	N†	Markedly Improved	Slightly Improved	Total Improved	No Change	Total Worsened
Under 40	Under 10	High	53	10 (19%)	10 (19%)	20 (38%)	23 (43%)	10 (19%)
		Low	46	3 (7%)	2 (4%)	5 (11%)‡	30 (65%)	11 (24%)
		Placebo	35	1 (3%)‡	3 (9%)	4 (11%)‡	9 (26%)	22 (63%)‡
		Routine	61	1 (2%)‡	9 (15%)	10 (16%)‡	41 (67%)	10 (16%)
Under 40	Over 10	High	23	1 (4%)	7 (30%)	8 (35%)	12 (52%)	3 (13%)
		Low	32	2 (6%)	3 (9%)	5 (16%)	18 (56%)	9 (28%)
		Placebo	24	0	1 (4%)	1 (4%)‡	6 (25%)	17 (71%)‡
		Routine	21	0	3 (14%)	3 (14%)	12 (57%)	6 (29%)
Over 40	Under 10	High	37	5 (13%)	8 (22%)	13 (35%)	19 (51%)	5 (14%)
		Low	33	5 (15%)	7 (21%)	12 (36%)	15 (45%)	6 (18%)
		Placebo	32	3 (9%)	2 (6%)	5 (16%)	15 (47%)	12 (38%)‡
		Routine	29	2 (7%)	9 (31%)	11 (38%)	17 (59%)	1 (3%)
Over 40	Over 10	High	78	4 (5%)	7 (9%)	11 (14%)	56 (72%)	11 (14%)
		Low	77	2 (3%)	10 (13%)	12 (16%)	52 (68%)	13 (17%)
		Placebo	98	1 (1%)	9 (9%)	10 (10%)	60 (61%)	28 (28%)‡
		Routine	83	3 (4%)	6 (7%)	9 (11%)	68 (82%)	6 (7%)

* Change in global psychiatric state is determined from the Global Improvement Scale comparing the patient's clinical condition at termination with his clinical condition prior to treatment.

† Data are presented only for patients who were evaluated by the same rater at pretreatment and termination.

‡ The difference between this group and the high dose group is significant at the $P = 0.05$ level (chi square analysis).

other treatments with this subgroup of patients. Chi-square analyses revealed that the high dose group had a significantly higher proportion of markedly improved patients than the routine treatment group and placebo group. The high dose also produced more marked improvement than the low dose group, but this approached significance only at the 0.1 level. When all degrees of improvement (slight plus marked) were included in the analysis, the high dose group showed a significantly higher incidence of improvement than each of the other treatments.

Younger, More Hospitalized Patients (Under 40, Hospitalized Over Ten Years).

This subgroup of patients also appeared to benefit from the high dose treatment. However, slight improvement accounted for practically all the difference between the high dose group and each of the other treatments. Marked improvement occurred in only 4% of the high dose patients.

Older, Less Hospitalized Patients (Over 40, Hospitalized Under Ten Years).

The greatest improvement on low dose and routine treatment occurred with this subgroup of patients. The high dose group also showed a high incidence of improvement with these patients, but did not differ significantly from the routine treatment and low dose groups.

Older, More Hospitalized Patients (Over 40, Hospitalized Over Ten Years).

The high dose treatment was least effective with this subgroup of patients. Only 14% of the high dose patients improved as compared to 16% of the low dose patients and 10% of the placebo patients.

There is one other noteworthy finding from the Global Scale. In the placebo group, clinical change was clearly a function of age: 66% of the patients under 40 were found to be worse, as contrasted with only 31% of the patients over 40.

Global Severity of Illness Scale

The covariance analyses of the Global Severity of Illness Scale showed that high dose was significantly more effective than low dose and routine treatment only with younger, less hospitalized patients. High dose was significantly more effective than placebo at all levels of age and hospitalization.

When pre-post change scores were tested for significance, it was found that the only significant improvement in global severity of illness occurred among younger, less hospitalized patients on high dose. Significant worsening occurred with the placebo group at all levels of age and hospitalization.

Despite the significant improvement effected in younger, less hospitalized, high dose patients, it might be asked to what extent these patients were still mentally ill after treatment. Table 3 gives the distribution of pretreatment and posttreatment scores on the Global Severity of Illness Scale. It may be observed that improvement in younger, less hospitalized patients consisted mainly of a shift from marked and moderate illness to mild and borderline illness: 25% were rated mildly or borderline mentally ill after treatment as compared to 6% prior to treatment.

Changes in Specific Symptoms and Behavior

The DRI, IMPS, and NOSIE provide measures of 21 specific symptoms and behaviors. The results from these three instruments correspond very closely to results from the Global Scales. Briefly, the results may be summarized as follows:

1. On all three scales, high dose was found to be the most effective treatment for younger, less hospitalized patients. Significant treatment differences for this subgroup of patients are shown in Table 4. It may be seen that high dose was significantly more effective than low dose and placebo in 18 of 21 symptom areas. High dose was significantly superior to routine treatment in nine areas, including the important DRI measures of Community Adjustment Potential and Psychosocial Adequacy. In no symptom area was high dose less effective than the other treatments.

Table 5 gives the difference between pre- and post-treatment scores for younger, less hospitalized patients. Significant difference scores are shown with an asterisk. High dose patients showed significant improvement of 15 of the 21 measures. Even on the other six measures, change was in the direction of improvement. The only other significant improvement occurred with routine treatment in the areas of Excitement (IMPS), Hostile–Belligerence (IMPS), Manifest Psychosis (NOSIE), and Paranoid Depression (NOSIE).

TABLE 3

Pretreatment and Posttreatment Ratings on the Global Severity of Illness Scale

Age in Years	Years Currently in Hospital	Treatment Group	N*	PRETREATMENT SEVERITY OF ILLNESS				POSTTREATMENT SEVERITY OF ILLNESS			
				Marked or Worse	Moderate	Mild	Borderline	Marked or Worse	Moderate	Mild	Borderline
Under 40	Under 10	High	53	70%	25%	6%	0	60%	15%	17%	8%
		Low	46	67%	28%	4%	0	78%	17%	4%	0
		Placebo	35	74%	23%	3%	0	91%	0	9%	0
		Routine	61	72%	15%	11%	2%	69%	18%	11%	2%
Under 40	Over 10	High	23	70%	17%	9%	4%	70%	22%	4%	4%
		Low	32	72%	25%	3%	0	78%	19%	3%	0
		Placebo	24	83%	17%	0	0	92%	8%	0	0
		Routine	21	90%	10%	0	0	90%	10%	0	0
Over 40	Under 10	High	37	70%	15%	11%	5%	57%	24%	14%	5%
		Low	33	55%	27%	12%	6%	52%	24%	17%	6%
		Placebo	32	59%	31%	10%	0	78%	12%	6%	3%
		Routine	29	58%	31%	5%	5%	45%	38%	12%	5%
Over 40	Over 10	High	78	83%	12%	5%	0	73%	21%	4%	1%
		Low	77	73%	25%	3%	0	74%	19%	7%	0
		Placebo	98	74%	18%	5%	2%	86%	11%	3%	1%
		Routine	83	82%	12%	6%	1%	92%	6%	2%	0

* Data are presented only for patients who were evaluated by the same rater at pretreatment and termination.

TABLE 4

DRI, IMPS, and NOSIE Measures*

Groups Being Compared	Measures Showing a Significant Difference Between Groups $(P < 0.05)$ †			
High dose group more improved than low dose group	Psychosocial Adequacy	(DRI)	Motor Disturbances	(IMPS)
	Belligerence‡	(DRI)	Conceptual Disorganization	(IMPS)
	Community Adjustment	(DRI)	Social Competence	(NOSIE)
	Manifest Psychopathology	(DRI)	Social Interest‡	(NOSIE)
	Excitement	(IMPS)	Cooperation	(NOSIE)
	Hostile-Belligerence‡	(IMPS)	Personal Neatness	(NOSIE)
	Paranoid Projection	(IMPS)	Irritability	(NOSIE)
	Perceptual Distortions	(IMPS)	Manifest Psychosis	(NOSIE)
	Disorientation	(IMPS)	Paranoid Depression	(NOSIE)
High dose group more improved than routine treatment group	Psychosocial Adequacy	(DRI)	Conceptual Disorganization	(IMPS)
	Community Adjustment	(DRI)	Social Competence	(NOSIE)
	Paranoid Projection	(IMPS)	Cooperation	(NOSIE)
	Disorientation	(IMPS)	Irritability	(NOSIE)
	Motor Disturbances	(IMPS)		
High dose group more improved than placebo	Psychosocial Adequacy	(DRI)	Motor Disturbances	(IMPS)
	Belligerence	(DRI)	Conceptual Disorganization	(IMPS)
	Community Adjustment	(DRI)	Social Competence	(NOSIE)
	Manifest Psychopathology	(DRI)	Social Interest	(NOSIE)
	Excitement	(IMPS)	Cooperation	(NOSIE)
	Hostile-Belligerence	(IMPS)	Personal Neatness	(NOSIE)
	Paranoid Projection	(IMPS)	Irritability	(NOSIE)
	Perceptual Distortions	(IMPS)	Manifest Psychosis	(NOSIE)
	Disorientation	(IMPS)	Paranoid Depression	(NOSIE)
High dose group less improved than any other treatment group	None			

* Showing a significant difference between high dose and low dose, high dose and routine treatment, and high dose and placebo for younger, less hospitalized patients. Younger, less hospitalized patients are patients under age 40 who have been hospitalized less than ten years.

† Treatment groups were compared by analysis of covariance which adjusts for pretreatment level.

‡ Difference significant only for female patients.

Placebo and low dose patients showed significant worsening or no change on all measures.

2. The results with high dose were less impressive among older patients and patients hospitalized over ten years. High dose was significantly superior to low dose and routine treatment in only five

TABLE 5

Difference Between Pretreatment and Posttreatment Means for Younger, Less Hospitalized Patients in Four Treatment Groups

Symptom or Behavior	MEAN DIFFERENCE SCORE			
	High	Low	Placebo	Routine
DRI				
Psychosocial Adequacy	+12.6*	−8.3	−34.6*	+0.5
Community Adjustment	+ 6.6*	−7.3*	−21.4*	−0.2
Belligerence	+ 2.1	−4.3*	− 8.0*	+1.2
Manifest Psychosis	+ 2.3*	−0.7	− 2.6*	+1.3
NOSIE				
Social Competence	+ 6.2*	−4.3	−18.9*	+1.3
Social Interest	+ 0.5	−8.7	−24.1*	−0.5
Personal Neatness	+ 3.0*	−2.5*	− 8.5*	−1.0
Cooperation	+ 3.7*	−4.6*	−12.1*	−0.8
Irritability	+ 8.5*	+5.0	−17.2*	+3.0
Manifest Psychosis	+ 4.7*	−1.0	− 9.1*	+2.4*
Paranoid Depression	+ 2.0*	−0.2	− 1.6*	+1.9*
IMPS				
Excitement	+ 7.4*	0.0	−16.0*	+5.8*
Hostile-Belligerence	+ 8.3*	−3.7	−13.7*	+6.0*
Paranoid Projection	+ 4.1*	−4.5	−11.3*	−1.6
Grandiose-Expansiveness	+ 0.2	−2.1	− 4.0	+2.0
Perceptual Distortions	+ 6.8*	−2.9	− 9.3*	+4.0
Anxious Intropunitiveness	+ 5.4	+3.9	− 0.2	+0.9
Retardation and Apathy	+ 1.4	−3.9	− 7.1	−2.9
Disorientation	+ 7.3*	−5.5	−19.5*	+0.6
Motor Disturbances	+ 4.7*	−1.0	−21.4*	+0.5
Conceptual Disorganization	+ 3.8	−1.6	−13.0*	+2.4

Younger, less hospitalized patients are patients under age 40 who have been hospitalized less than ten years.

Mean Difference Score: A "plus" difference indicates improvement from pretreatment to posttreatment, and a "minus" difference indicates worsening.

* Difference score significant at $P = 0.05$.

symptom areas: Excitement (IMPS), Paranoid Projection (IMPS), Conceptual Disorganization (IMPS), Motor Disturbance (IMPS), and Irritability (NOSIE). High dose was significantly more effective than placebo in most symptom areas. However, this was due more to placebo worsening than to high dose improvement.

3. Routine treatment was particularly effective with patients over 40 having less than ten years of hospitalization. With this subgroup of patients, routine treatment was significantly better than high dose in several important areas, including Community Adjustment Potential (DRI), Psychosocial Adequacy (DRI), Social Competence (NOSIE), and Retardation and Apathy (IMPS).

4. The results on Retardation and Apathy deserve special mention. Based on the chlorpromazine literature, the expectation was that high dose would be less effective than the other treatments in reducing symptoms measured by this factor—ie, slowed motor behavior, reduced general reactivity, and apathy. It was therefore surprising to find that with younger, less hospitalized patients, high dose actually reduced Retardation and Apathy more than the other treatments (although the difference between high dose and the other treatments was significant at only the 0.1 level). At the other levels of age and hospitalization, the results with high dose were consistent with the literature: high dose showed a significant increase in Retardation and Apathy and was the least effective of the four treatments.

Time of Improvement

Preliminary analysis of the trends of clinical change over the six-month treatment period indicated that most high dose patients reached a plateau of improvement by four months. Patients on low dose generally achieved maximum improvement within two months; the greatest deterioration on placebo occurred during the third and fourth months of the study. The routine treatment group showed no clear pattern of change. Clinical change on routine treatment was highly variable. Some patients who showed improvement at two months were deteriorated at six months, and vice versa.

Early Terminations

Table 6 shows the number of patients in each treatment group who were dropped from the study because of side effects or deteriorated behavior. The placebo group had the highest percentage of drop-outs (38%), followed by the high dose group (25%), and the low

TABLE 6
Percent of Treatment-Related Terminations in Three Treatment Groups

Reason for Termination	TREATMENT GROUP		
	High (N = 208) %	Low (N = 208) %	Placebo (N = 212) %
Side effects			
Cardiovascular	6	1	1
Neurological	3	0	0
Ophthalmologic	7	1	1
Weight loss	1	0	2
Other	2	1	1
Total side effects	20	2	5
Deteriorated behavior	5	13	33
Total terminations	25	15	38

dose group (15%). Terminations because of side effects were most frequent with the high dose group, but the placebo group had the highest incidence of dropouts due to deteriorated behavior. In addition to the terminations listed in Table 6, approximately 3% of the high dose patients and 2% of the low dose patients went home on trial visit; another 4% to 6% of the patients in each treatment group were terminated for administrative reasons.

Time of Early Termination

Of the 51 high dose patients dropped from the study, 25% were terminated during the first eight weeks, 45% during the second eight weeks, and 30% during the last eight weeks. The time pattern of dropouts for the placebo group was similar to that for the high dose group. Of the 82 placebo dropouts, 24% occurred during the first eight weeks, 56% during the second eight weeks, and 20% during the last eight weeks. The 31 low dose dropouts were evenly distributed across the three eight-week periods. Time of termination was not related to sex, age, or length of hospitalization in any of the three treatment groups.

Side Effects

Table 7 presents the incidence of side effects judged to be moderate or severe in each study treatment. The high dose group had the highest percentage of patients with at least one moderate to severe side effect (61%), followed by the placebo group (41%), low dose group (34%), and routine treatment group (15%). The side effects showing the greatest difference between groups are listed below:

Eye Change. Only a brief description of eye change will be presented here. A more detailed report is presented in another paper.[16] Ocular change occurred in 35% of the high dose group, 12% of the low dose group, 8% of the placebo group, and 5% of the routine treatment group. As can be observed in Table 7, the distribution of stellate (grade 2) lens opacities was approximately the same for the four treatment groups. Disciform (grade 1) lens opacities, however, occurred much more frequently in the high dose group. A surprising finding was the occurrence of anterior corneal change in 26% of the high dose group. This change sometimes appeared as diffuse bedewing, usually whitish but occasionally brownish. The change usually appeared only in the inferior two thirds of the cornea and was often identical in appearance with corneal change seen with chloroquine toxicity. There is ample evidence that the change is reversible. At nine months after conclusion of the study, approximately 50% of the corneal opacities had improved markedly or disappeared completely. There was no report of reduction in visual acuity that could be attributed to either lenticular or corneal changes.

Photosensitivity Reactions. More than 20% of the patients in the high dose group had photosensitivity reactions, as compared to 2% of the patients in the other treatment groups. There was a significant relationship between photosensitivity reactions and eye changes in the high dose group. Approximately 75% of the patients with photosensitivity reactions developed eye opacities, in contrast to only 24% with out photosensitivity reactions.

Cardiovascular Effects. Moderate to severe cardiovascular reactions (dizziness, syncope, hypotension) occurred in 26% of the high dose patients, 9% of the low dose patients, and 8% of the placebo patients. Cardiovascular side effects were particularly se-

TABLE 7

Percent of Patients in Each Treatment Group
With Side Effects of at Least Moderate Severity

	TREATMENT GROUP			
Side Effect*	High (N = 208) %	Low (N = 208) %	Placebo (N = 212) %	Routine (N = 213) %
Central Nervous System				
Akathisia	9	9	16	5
Dystonic reaction	9	1	2	0
Parkinson reaction	16	8	13	5
Seizures	6	1	0	0
Autonomic Nervous System				
Dizziness, faintness	19	6	7	1
Syncope	2	1	2	1
Dry mouth	9	2	1	1
Nasal congestion	1	1	1	0
Constipation	7	2	3	1
Diarrhea	2	1	1	0
Urinary disturbance	2	1	1	0
Nausea, vomiting	3	2	3	1
Salivation	5	1	1	0
Allergic Reactions				
Rashes, itching	7	1	5	1
Photosensitivity	22	2	2	1
Other				
Drowsiness	38	15	14	6
Peripheral edema	3	1	1	0
Blurred vision	1	0	1	0
Eye opacities				
Lens-grade 1†	19	7	5	2
Lens-grade 2	2	4	2	3
Anterior cornea	26	1	1	1
Total with opacities	35	12	8	5
Side effects requiring antiparkinson medication	31	12	12	27

* Refers either to adverse reactions which occurred for the first time during treatment or to reactions which became more severe after treatment was started.

† Opacities disciform in shape with no accumulation along the sutures were classified as grade 1. Stellate shaped opacities were classified as grade 2.

vere in older women on high dose medication. Approximately 14% of the high dose women over 40 were terminated for cardiovascular disturbances; another 21% had their dose reduced at some time during the study to control for severe cardiovascular symptoms.

Seizures. Twelve patients had a total of 17 convulsive seizures during the treatment period. Eleven of these patients were in the high dose group and one was in the low dose group.

Drowsiness. Excessive drowsiness was the most common side effect in the high dose group, occurring in 38% of the patients. Drowsiness was most severe during the first three weeks on maximum dose. When severe drowsiness persisted, reduction of the 2,000 mg dose to 1,500 or 1,600 mg generally reduced the drowsiness to a tolerable level.

Extrapyramidal Reactions. The high dose group had the highest incidence of dystonic reactions and Parkinson-like symptoms (tremor, rigidity), and the placebo group had the highest incidence of what was reported as akathisia. Although the incidence of akathisia and parkinsonism did not differ greatly among high, low, and placebo groups, the reactions occurring with high dose patients were often more severe and required more extensive use of antiparkinsonian medication. Thirty-one percent of the high dose patients, 12% of the low dose patients, and 12% of the placebo

TABLE 8

Percent of Improved and Unimproved High Dose Patients Having No Moderate to Severe Side Effects*

| | | PERCENT WITH NO SERIOUS SIDE EFFECTS | | |
| | | --- | --- | --- |
Age in Years	Years Currently in Hospital	Improved Patients %	Unimproved Patients %	Total Patients %
Under 40	Under 10	45	48	47
Under 40	Over 10	50	47	49
Over 40	Under 10	46	33	38
Over 40	Over 10	36	30	31

* Based on Global Improvement Scale.

patients received antiparkinsonian medication at some time during the study. It should be noted, however, that the percentage of high dose patients on antiparkinsonian medication did not differ significantly from the percentage of routine treatment patients receiving antiparkinsonian drugs during the treatment period (see Table 7). In addition to the above side effects, dry mouth, excessive salivation, constipation, and rashes also occurred most frequently in the high dose group.

One death occurred during the course of treatment. The patient was a 37-year-old woman on 1,700 mg of chlorpromazine. The patient died after a grand mal seizure, reported to be the third seizure in a three-hour period. Autopsy findings were essentially normal. Ventricular fibrillation during a convulsive seizure is a possible explanation.

Side Effects by Age and Sex. A detailed report of side effects in various age and sex groups will be presented in a future paper. Briefly, the relationship between treatment age, and sex may be summarized as follows: In the high dose group, the greatest frequency and severity of side effects occurred in older women, followed by older men, younger men, and younger women, in that order. In the placebo group, younger patients, particularly men, had the highest incidence of moderate to severe reactions, whereas in the low dose group and routine treatment group there was no apparent sex or age effect.

Dosage Reduction. There were 146 high dose patients (70% of the total sample) who completed the full 24 weeks of treatment. Of these, 108 (75%) were on the maximum dose of 2,000 mg at the end of the study. Only 12 patients finished the study on doses below 1,600 mg. Cardiovascular disturbance, particularly in older women, was the principal cause of dose reduction.

Occurrence of Side Effects and Clinical Change. There was no apparent relationship between occurrence of side effects and clinical improvement. Table 8 gives the percent of improved and unimproved high dose patients who had no moderate to severe side effects. The criteria for improvement used in this table was the Global Improvement Scale. The other scales provided similar results.

COMMENT

The results indicate that high dose is significantly more effective than low dose, placebo, and routine treatment with younger, less hospitalized patients (ie, patients under 40 with less than ten years current hospitalization). With older or longer hospitalized patients, high dose appears to offer no great advantage over low dose and routine treatment.

The range of symptoms affected by high dose chlorpromazine among younger, less hospitalized patients was impressive. There was significant improvement in 15 of the 21 symptom areas measured by the IMPS, DRI, and NOSIE. Even in the other six symptom areas, change (though nonsignificant) was in the direction of improvement. This wide range of improvement suggests that the effectiveness of high doses extends beyond mere "tranquilization" or sedation. In particular, the improvement in the key schizophrenic areas of delusional thinking, hallucinations, and disorientation suggests that high dose chlorpromazine is an effective antipsychotic treatment with younger, less hospitalized patients.

A basic question that may be asked of all drug studies reporting symptomatic improvement among chronic schizophrenics is whether the treatment has resulted in improvement in practical aspects of the patient's adjustment, namely those areas of behavior that most affect the patient's ability to leave the hospital and adjust in the community. Our results indicate that younger, less hospitalized patients on high dose, in addition to showing generalized symptom reduction, also show significant improvement in areas of social adjustment known to be related to release. This improvement is particularly meaningful, since the areas of change—Psychosocial Adequacy and Community Adjustment Potential—represent the most characteristic features of discharge-ready patients. What remains to be answered is whether or not these improved patients are in fact able to leave the hospital. Further analyses are planned to determine the extent to which improved study patients resemble the discharge-ready patients seen in the DRI validation study.

These findings, however, do not justify a blanket endorsement of high dose treatment for all younger, less hospitalized patients. Approximately one fifth of the population of schizophrenics under 40 hospitalized less than ten years were screened from the study prior to treatment because of medical conditions contraindicating the use of high doses of chlorpromazine. Even with the "clean" sample used in the study, approximately half the patients had at least one moderate to severe side effect during treatment. Ten percent showed side effects serious enough to warrant termination from the study. Thus, high dose treatment is not undertaken without some risk. However, the fact that 45% of the younger, less hospitalized patients showing improvement had no moderate to severe side effects indicates that high dose can be both safe and clinically effective. Hopefully, further refinements of study data will provide greater sensitivity in describing the characteristics of patients for whom high dose chlorpromazine is the appropriate treatment regimen.

Among older or longer hospitalized patients, high dose was more effective than low dose and routine treatment in a number of symptom areas (including Paranoid Projection, Conceptual Disorganization, Motor Disturbance, and Irritability). Despite this symptomatic improvement, high dose showed no significant superiority over low dose and routine treatment on either the Global Scales or the important DRI factors of Community Adjustment Potential and Psychosocial Adequacy. In light of this, it is doubtful whether the clinical benefits of high dose with older or longer hospitalized patients justify the high risk of side effects. This is particularly true with older patients, where the risk of side effects is greatest.

One interesting finding was that patients hospitalized under ten years had significantly more florid symptomatology (ie, perceptual, delusional, and conceptual disturbance) and showed significantly more social competence than patients hospitalized over ten years. This finding supports a theory often advanced by the proponents of social psychiatry. It is argued that the acute psychotic symptoms that characterize the early stages of schizophrenic illness subside over time,[17] only to be replaced by deficiencies in social competence fostered by the "total institution."[18-22] Lack of contact with the community, minimal challenge to social and interpersonal skills, and the "custodial" atmosphere of the chronic ward all contribute to this progressive deterioration. (Other tenable explanations are the existence of a progressive "organic" impairment of brain function or selection release of less impaired members of the chronic schizophrenic population.) The result is that patients hospitalized for long periods of time may suffer more from the debilitating effects of "institutionalization" than from the primary effects of the schizophrenic illness. This could explain why only a few of the study patients hospitalized more than ten years showed marked improvement. It may be unreasonable to expect phenothiazine therapies to undo the effects of many years of social deprivation and provide the patients with the social and personal resources that they lack.

This study leaves no doubt that chlorpromazine side effects are related to both dose and age. High dose produced more frequent and serious side effects than low dose at all levels of age and hospitalization. Among patients on high dose, older patients, particularly women, showed more severe cardiovascular reaction, drowsiness, and parkinsonism than younger patients. The incidence of side effects was not related to length of hospitalization or weight. There was also no significant relationship between occurrence of side effects and clinical improvement.

The results on placebo present a mixed picture. On the doctors' interview scales, the majority of older patients on placebo showed no measurable deterioration over the six-month study period. On the ward, the results were far less positive. The nurses rated the majority of older placebo patients as worse in most symptom areas. The most likely explanation for this discrepancy between interview and ward findings is that the nurses, who were continually exposed to the patient on the ward, were more sensitive to signs of behavioral deterioration than the interview rater, who saw the patient only once every two months. The social workers, who also had extensive contact with the patients on the ward, described the older patients as consistently worse in most symptom areas. Only 26% of the older placebo patients were actually withdrawn from the study because of deteriorated behavior. However, a sizable number of patients remaining in the study showed noticeable regression on the ward, and it is doubtful that they would have remained off medication had they not been involved in a study. Even if the relapse rate of 26% is taken at face value, it would still seem too high to justify long-term drug withdrawal as a treatment policy with older schizophrenic patients.

Some investigators advocate treatment programs for chronic patients that involve periodic short-term withdrawal of phenothiazine medication.[23-25] Although this study was not designed to evaluate the effectiveness of these "intermittent chemotherapy" programs, our placebo results do indicate that when such programs are used, the drug-free period should not exceed two months. After this period, the probability of relapse and deterioration sharply increases.

The treatment prescribed by the hospital physician (ie, routine treatment) was most effective with patients over 40 having less than ten years' hospitalization. Most of the study patients benefiting from routine treatment had been initially hospitalized late in life (ie, after age 30). Many showed cyclic patterns of illness, and had been discharged a number of times prior to the study.

Results from the routine treatment group should be interpreted with a certain amount of caution. Ward evaluations were not done under double-blind conditions. The research nurses supervised the administration of study medication and were thus aware which patients were in the routine treatment group. Patients in the routine treatment group were also known to the physicians evaluating the side effects. Despite those limitations, the routine treatment group was a highly valuable control group that allowed us to compare study treatments with treatments the physicians considered best for the patient.

There was no difference between treatment groups in the number of patients actually leaving the hospital. Only a few patients in each treatment group (2% to 4%) were discharged or granted a trial visit during or immediately following treatment. It is questionable, however, whether discharge can be regarded as a meaningful criterion of improvement. It has been argued that hospital and community deficiencies are often more important than clinical condition in keeping the schizophrenic patient in the hospital.[26] The success or failure of discharge seems to be particularly dependent on the relationship between the chronic patient and his family or other key figures in the community.[27] It is apparent that drug effectiveness cannot be measured by discharge rate if this, in turn, is significantly influenced by such indirect criteria. The use of valid and reliable rating instruments such as the DRI and IMPS appears to be the best method available for evaluating effects of psychopharmacologic agents in chronic schizophrenic patients.

SUMMARY

In a collaborative study involving 838 chronic schizophrenics in seven public mental hospitals, a high dose regimen of chlorpromazine (2,000 mg/day) was compared with a low dose chlorpromazine regimen (300 mg/day), a placebo, and routine hospital treatment. Treatment followed a double-blind procedure for 24 weeks. Clinical evaluations using five rating scales provided 23 criteria of change. The following results were obtained:

1. High dose was significantly more effective than low dose, placebo, and routine treatment with patients under 40 currently hospitalized less than ten years. High dose improvement with younger, less hospitalized patients included change in a wide range of schizophrenic symptoms and behaviors. Particularly significant was the improvement in Psychosocial Adequacy and Community Adjustment Potential—two areas of social adjustment known to be related to release.

2. Among older or longer hospitalized patients, high dose appeared to offer no great advantage over low dose or routine treatment.

3. High dose produced a significantly greater number of serious side effects than each of the other treatments. Side effects from high dose were particularly severe in older patients (ie, over 40 years of age).

4. Placebo patients showed significant worsening on practically all criteria of change. Greatest deterioration occurred during the third and fourth months of treatment.

5. Routine treatment was most effective among patients over 40 with less than ten years hospitalization.

Additional analyses relating to prediction of outcome on high dose and placebo are in progress.

REFERENCES

1. Ayd, F.: Large Doses of Chlorpromazine in Treatment of Psychiatric Patients, *Dis. Nerv. Syst.*, 16:146–149, 1955.
2. Delay, J., and Deniker, P.: Chlorpromazine and Neuroleptic Treatments in Psychiatry, *J. Clin. Exp. Psychopath.*, 17:19–24, 1956.
3. Forrest, F., et al: Drug Maintenance Problems of Rehabilitated Mental Patients: Current Drug-Dosage "Merry-Go-Round," *Amer. J. Psychiat.*, 121:33–40, 1964.
4. Kinross-Wright, V.: Intensive Chlorpromazine Treatment of Schizophrenia, *Psychiat. Res. Rep. Amer. Psychiat. Assoc.*, 1:53–62, 1955.
5. Lieberman, D.: Tranquilizers in Psychiatry: Chlorpromazine Therapy, *Brit. Med. J.*, 1:512–513, 1956.
6. Mendelsohn, R., Penmon, A., and Schiele, B.: Massive Chlorpromazine Therapy, *Psychiat. Quart.*, 33:55–76, 1959.
7. Pollack, B.: Preliminary Report on 500 Patients Treated with Thorazine at Rochester State Hospital, *Psychiat. Quart.*, 29:439–456, 1955.
8. Rosati, D.: Prolonged High Dosage Ataractic Medication in Chronic Schizophrenia, *Brit. J. Psychiat.*, 110:61–63, 1964.
9. Schiele, B., et al: Comparison of Low and High Dosage Procedures in Chlorpromazine Therapy, *Psychiat. Quart.*, 33:252–259, 1959.
10. Winkleman, W.: Clinical and Socio-Cultural Study of 200 Psychiatric Pa-

tients Started on Chlorpromazine 10½ Years Ago, *Amer. J. Psychiat.*, 120: 861–869, 1964.
11. Hogarty, G.: Discharge Readiness: Components of a Casework Judgment, *Soc. Casework*, 47:165–171, 1966.
12. Hogarty, G.: Discharge Readiness Inventory: Validity as Outcome Measure in Treatment of Chronic Schizophrenia, read before the Fifth Annual Meeting of the American College of Neuropsychopharmacology, San Juan, P.R., 1966.
13. Lorr, M., et al: *Inpatient Multidimensional Psychiatric Scale: Manual,* Palo Alto, Calif.: Consulting Psychologist Press, 1962.
14. Honigfeld, G., and Klett, C.: Nurse's Observation Scale for Inpatient Evaluation (NOSIE): New Scale for Measuring Improvement in Chronic Schizophrenia, *J. Clin. Psychol.*, 21:65–71, 1965.
15. Winer, B. J.: *Statistical Principles in Experimental Design,* New York: McGraw-Hill Book Co., Inc., 1962.
16. Delong, S., Prien, R., and Cole, J.: Opacities During Prolonged High Dose Chlorpromazine Therapy, *Arch. Ophthal.*, to be published.
17. Casey, J., et al: Combined Drug Treatment of Chronic Schizophrenia, *Amer. J. Psychiat.*, 117:997–1002, 1961.
18. Barton, R.: *Institutional Neurosis,* Bristol, England: John Wright & Sons, Ltd., 1959.
19. Brown, G., and Wing, J.: Comparative Clinical and Social Survey of Three Mental Hospitals, *Sociol. Rev.* [Monogr.], No. 5, 1962.
20. Goffman, E.: *Asylums: Essays on Social Situation of Mental Patients and Other Inmates,* New York: Doubleday & Co., Inc., 1961.
21. Martin, D.: Institutionalization, *Lancet,* 2:1188–1192, 1955.
22. Stanton, A., and Schwartz, N.: *The Mental Hospital: A Study of Institutional Participation in Psychiatric Illness and Treatment,* New York: Basic Books, 1954.
23. Good, W., Sterling, M., and Holtzman, W.: Termination of Chlorpromazine with Schizophrenic Patients, *Amer. J. Psychiat.*, 115:443–448, 1959.
24. Olson, G., and Peterson, D.: Sudden Removal of Tranquilizing Drugs from Chronic Psychiatric Patients, *J. Nerv. Ment. Dis.*, 131:252–255, 1960.
25. Rothstein, C.: Evaluation of Effects of Discontinuation of Chlorpromazine, *New Eng. J. Med.*, 2:67–69, 1960.
26. Hogarty, G.: Hospital Differences in Retention and Release of "Discharge-Ready" Chronic Schizophrenics, Special Studies Section, Psychopharmacology Research Branch, NIMH. Prepublication report.
27. Gordon, H., and Groth, C.: Mental Patients Wanting to Stay in Hospital: Attitudes, *Arch. Gen. Psychiat.*, 4:124–130, 1961.

9

*Depot Fluphenazine Facilitation of Treatment of Psychosis**

by JOVAN SIMEON,

ALI KESKINER, MAX FINK,

and TURAN M. ITIL

This chapter concerning the intramuscular use of fluphenazine decanoate at monthly and bimonthly intervals is one of timely importance. A well-designed scientific exploration of depot fluphenazine, this study shows its psychopharmacologic effectiveness as a phenothiazine and demonstrates the specific items of schizophrenia it helps to relieve. The study findings offer an optimistic probability that this drug will bring widespread relief to a multitude of patients not usually capable of following their aftercare treatment. Its practical advantage for use in community care will help to implement programs at present considered impractical and will facilitate a broader use in home care. This well-planned investigation deserves consideration for a more widespread application and replication.

Following discharge to the community, many improved psychotic patients require rehospitalization,[1] with relapse often being related

* Aided, in part, by USPHS MH-11381 and 13358, this report summarizes studies in progress since 1965 that have been published in part (12,13).

We are indebted to Drs. Luigi Bucci, Maria Fuchs, and J. M. C. Holden for their participation in these studies, and to Dr. Alain Sanseigne of Squibb Institute for Medical Research for making supplies of fluphenazine enanthate and decanoate freely available.

to an inadequate drug intake or its discontinuation.[2-4] Sustained improvement of discharged patients depends on the maintenance of psychotropic drug treatment for prolonged periods.[5-7] When the initiative for drug intake passes from the nurse to the patient or his family, drug intake may cease because of a sense of well-being, poor insight and judgment, delusions, fear, neglect, failure to keep appointments, miscalculations of dosage, or expense.[2, 4] The necessity for frequent daily ingestions represents a chore, and even non-psychiatric patients neglect their treatment under similar conditions.

The development of depot fluphenazines—potent antipsychotic drugs with long duration of action—offers an effective way to prevent recidivism, and a greater convenience and better control of drug administration by the therapist.

Fluphenazine has the broad therapeutic spectrum similar to that of piperazine phenothiazines. It has a wide safety margin, for it has been effectively used in oral daily dosages from 5 to 1200 mg without disabling secondary or extrapyramidal symptoms.[8] Interestingly, in high dosages, the extrapyramidal effects are less marked than at lower dosages. Above 800 mg antiparkinson medication was discontinued, only to be needed again when dosages were reduced.[8]

Two depot forms of fluphenazine, the enanthate and the decanoate, have been tested and are available in vials of 10 cc containing 25 mg/cc.

In animal studies, depot forms produce a more uniform effect at a considerably lower total dose than daily administrations of fluphenazine hydrochloride. Fluphenazine decanoate (FD) has the same spectrum of activity, but a slower onset, a lower initial peak, and a longer duration of action than fluphenazine enanthate (FE) in the conditioned avoidance inhibition tests in rats and dogs.[9]

Clinical studies of FE demonstrated the efficacy of single intramuscular injections for 7 to 21 days in maintaining the improvement of severely psychotic patients.[10-18, 19, 20, 28] In 501 patients treated with FD, 47.1% responded better to FD than they did to previous phenothiazine therapy, suggesting that many psychiatric patients may not have taken their medication.[9]

The degree and incidence of parkinsonism, akathisia, and dystonia with the depot forms are similar to those with oral piperazine phenothiazines, and largely depend on whether antiparkinson drugs are administered concurrently. The successful use of depot fluphenazine requires the continued daily intake of antiparkinson drugs, and though this represents a drawback to therapy, it is minimized by the education of patients and their willingness to take this medication when the physical symptoms become manifest.

We have undertaken four studies of depot fluphenazines in severely ill psychotic patients to determine their duration of efficacy and whether FD and FE can substitute for other antipsychotic drugs as maintenance treatment.

FLUPHENAZINE DECANOATE IN CHRONIC PSYCHOSIS

A study was undertaken to determine the antipsychotic potency of FD and its ability to substitute for other psychotropic drugs as maintenance therapy.[21] Twenty-four psychotic inpatients were divided into two matched groups. Before FD was given, one group received placebo for 4 to 20 weeks (mean, 9 weeks), and the second, various psychotropic drugs for 4 to 96 weeks (mean, 18 weeks).

The initial doses of FD were given intramuscularly at weekly intervals, with the amount related to each patient's tolerance of previous piperazine phenothiazine drugs. Three patients received 12.5 mg; fourteen, 25 mg; and seven, 50 mg. The maintenance dose and frequency of injections depended on the clinical response, varying from 12.5 to 75 mg in one- to three-week intervals. Most patients received 25 to 50 mg weekly. Oral procyclidine or parenteral benztropine was given whenever extrapyramidal symptoms developed.

The minimum treatment period was 12 weeks in 6 patients and 24 weeks in 17. In one patient FD was discontinued after eight weeks because of persistent psychotic behavior and extrapyramidal symptoms. Global improvement was marked in five patients, moderate in nine, slight in four, none in five, and one was worse. Thirteen patients returned home, and four were dischargeable.

Clinical evaluations were made every two weeks using an 85-symptom rating scale, reflecting eleven symptom clusters.[22] A cumulative analysis[23] of symptoms before treatment and after 2 and 12 weeks showed a significant improvement, especially after two weeks (Figure 1).

Improvement was greatest in disorders of affect, person, thought process and content, volition, perception, motor behavior, and higher mental functions. Extrapyramidal symptoms with FD were similar to those seen with other piperazine phenothiazines. Increased alertness and feelings of weakness were common early in

Fig. 1: Group Psychopathological Cumulative Analysis

The numbers 5, 9, 21, etc., in the abscissa refer to the items in the psycho-pathological symptom rating scale. The symptom clusters contain varying numbers of items.

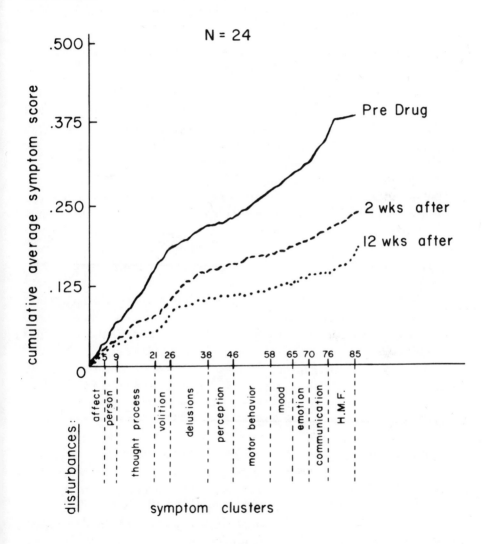

Reprinted from *Archives of General Psychiatry*, 18: 1968, with permission.

treatment. Of 14 female patients, menstruation ceased in seven and became irregular in two during treatment. In seven of these, such disturbances were seen with other phenothiazine drugs. Weight gain was not related to therapeutic outcome.

Changes in laboratory tests, blood pressure, and EKG were no greater than in control periods and populations.[24] There were no local or general complications due to intramuscular injections.

MAINTENANCE FLUPHENAZINE DECANOATE IN DISCHARGED PATIENTS

In the second study we determined the need for continued medication in chronic schizophrenic outpatients, and the efficacy of FD at fixed intervals to maintain their improvement.[25] Twenty-four patients, 20 female and four male, 22 to 50 years old (mean, 36), were included in the study. They had histories of 5 to 25 years (mean, 12.4 years) of mental illness, had been discharged from psychiatric inpatient services for six months to over three years (mean, 1.5 years), and had received antipsychotic drugs for up to 3½ years (mean, 2 years).

To establish a common baseline treatment response for all subjects, oral fluphenazine hydrochloride was given daily for six weeks, and all patients showed further improvement. The patients were randomly assigned into one group of 13 patients for FD treatment, and another of 11 patients for placebo. Both FD and placebo were given by intramuscular injection once every two weeks. If symptoms recurred by the time the next placebo injection was due, FD (25 mg) was given. Further dosages and intervals were individually adjusted. Antiparkinson drugs were given whenever necessary. Clinical assessments were made every two weeks, using global, psychopathologic, and psychosomatic rating scales.[22]

All 24 patients completed 12 weeks of FD or placebo injections. The average dose of FD was 28 to 32 mg every second week. Relapse was shown by three patients, one of whom was rehospitalized. In the placebo group, two patients relapsed within the first week, three by the fourth, and four by the sixth. Each of these nine patients received FD as soon as relapse was determined. Despite higher doses (to 75 mg) at shorter intervals, two patients were readmitted. Only three patients maintained their improvement on placebo, and these relapsed within six months.

A cumulative symptom analysis[23] showed that prior to treatment, the FD-treated patients had more psychopathology than the place-bo-treated patients. At the fourth week of parenteral treatment, the FD group showed further improvement, whereas the placebo group exhibited a recurrence of many of the principal symptoms of psychosis. By the 12th week, both group scores were similar, but for the placebo group the ratings showed less improvement than with oral fluphenazine, indicating that even a short interruption of drug treatment was accompanied by relapse and the symptoms difficult to relieve with retreatment.

The incidence of extrapyramidal symptoms during FD was equal to that during oral fluphenazine. There were no physical complications or laboratory abnormalities during the study.

FD-FE CROSSOVER IN AN AMBULATORY PSYCHOTIC POPULATION

The third study was undertaken to determine the efficacy of long-acting depot fluphenazine in the treatment and management of schizophrenic patients in a community mental health center, and to compare the relative value of fluphenazine decanoate and fluphenazine enanthate.[26] From a large population of outpatients considered treatment failures, 62 schizophrenic patients were included in the study. They ranged in age from 22 to 62 years (mean, 26.7), and two thirds were female. Every patient but one had a history of at least two years of mental illness.

Early in the study, dosages varied from 0.5 to 3 cc weekly. Later, the dosages of either drug were limited to 0.5 cc initially and 1.0 cc at weekly intervals until the third injection. Thereafter, the intervals were increased from two to four weeks, depending on the patient's response. Intervals of three weeks between injections of 1.0 cc were sufficient to maintain the improvement of many patients. Every patient was given antiparkinson drugs.

Twenty-two patients did not complete the crossover, with six improving before the treatment was discontinued.

The average dose remained fairly constant, but the intervals between injections generally increased more for FD than FE. The increase in time between injections was associated with persistence in symptomatic improvement.

Of 40 patients in the crossover, improvement was marked in 15, moderate in 20, and absent in 5. There were no differences in efficacy between FD and FE.

Extrapyramidal symptoms, if they occurred, usually appeared during the first three injections, and responded to antiparkinson drugs. Because of a higher starting dosage of FD, there was an apparent difference in efficacy and secondary effects between the two compounds.

FE-FD COMPARISON IN PRIOR-HOSPITALIZED SCHIZOPHRENIC OUTPATIENTS

The efficacy, tolerance, and duration of action of FD and FE were studied in chronic schizophrenic outpatients.[27]

Eighteen patients, 15 female and three male, 26 to 51 years old (mean 35.5), with mental illness of 6- to 26-year duration had been treated for 1.6 to 4 years (mean, 2.2) since discharge from the hospital prior to the study. The patients first received oral fluphenazine for six weeks, and then FD 2.5 to 75 mg every two weeks for 12 to 48 weeks (mean, 42). FE was then substituted for FD at equal dosage and intervals. Subsequent dosage changes depended on a patient's clinical condition. Antiparkinson drugs were maintained whenever required. FE was given for a minimum of 12 weeks, but after the eighth week, some patients received the drug at their homes from the research nurse.

During the first eight weeks of FE treatment, the dose had to be increased in three of five patients who felt the drug effects did not last until the next injection was due, and one required temporary hospitalization.

Because of a slight increase of the incidence and severity of akathisia and muscle rigidity, procyclidine had to be increased in two patients, and administered to another two who did not require antiparkinson drugs while receiving FD.

Statistical analysis of the global behavior and psychopathologic ratings[22] did not reveal significant differences between FD and FE.

On inquiry, patients were equally divided in their preference for the daily oral treatment and the depot parenteral one. Those objecting to the latter disliked receiving injections and the frequent hospital visits. Fourteen patients, however, preferred the depot treatment if given at home by a nurse, with hospital follow-up once every two or three months.

DISCUSSION

These studies confirm other reports[10-20] and establish the depot fluphenazines as effective antipsychotic drugs with single 25–50 mg intramuscular injections persisting in clinical efficacy for 7 to 28 days.[21, 25-27] Clinical efficacy was also apparent without prior oral phenothiazine therapy.

Depot fluphenazines can replace daily phenothiazine use in psychotic patients who require maintenance therapy. In such patients, dropout and rehospitalization rates are reduced. The obvious advantage of long-acting drugs is illustrated by the high rate of relapse when treatment is even briefly interrupted: 73% of schizophrenics showed psychotic regressions within six weeks, and 100% within six months, when they received placebo instead of drugs.[25] In addition, after six weeks of retreatment, prior levels of improvement were not achieved, indicating the risk of irregular medication. These long-acting antipsychotic drugs are also useful in the initial and custodial treatment of paranoid, uncooperative and negativistic inpatients, and in the maintenance of such patients in the community.

Further advantages in using depot fluphenazine result from the continued therapist-patient interaction, the introduction of regularity in the patient's observation and treatment increasing his confidence in the therapist. It also provides the basis for follow-up and special aftercare, and avoids the expense and nuisance of continued oral intake.

The safety margin of FE is illustrated by the use of 10 cc (250 mg) in single doses, with even fewer extrapyramidal symptoms than with dosages recommended in the United States.[27] No local inflammation or general physical complications have resulted from the intramuscular injections. The degree and incidence of extrapyramidal effects with depot fluphenazines are about equal to those seen with oral piperazine phenothiazines. It becomes necessary to administer antiparkinson drugs daily, preferably from the outset. Preventing parkinsonism is obviously better than treating it once it becomes manifest. Implicit in these studies is the importance of instructing and educating the patient and his family in the use of antiparkinson drugs.

For general clinical purposes, the enanthate and decanoate forms of fluphenazine have similar dosage and duration characteristics, although our studies and those of others suggest that the decanoate form may be associated with a longer duration of effect and fewer side reactions than the enanthate.

The majority of patients accept parenteral treatment with depot drugs. Though some patients object because they dislike injections and frequent visits to the hospital, very few refuse treatment. These objections can be further minimized if treatment is provided by a visiting nurse or the family physician.

It is our impression that the advent of long-acting psychotropic drugs represents a substantial improvement in the armamentarium of psychiatric therapies.

SUMMARY

Studies of depot fluphenazines—fluphenazine enanthate and decanoate—over a three-year period were undertaken in psychotic patients in two institutions. The data indicate that depot fluphenazine facilitates the treatment of psychosis and prevents relapse by ensuring regular drug administration and making its maintenance easier.

The proper application of this therapy requires initial dosages of 0.5 cc at 10- to 14-day intervals. The maintenance dosage is 0.5 to 1.5 cc every two to four weeks. Antiparkinson medication should be started in all patients at the onset of treatment.

The comparison of FD and FE indicates equivalent therapeutic efficacy, with a suggestion that FD may have a longer duration of action.

REFERENCES

1. Itil, T., Keskiner, A., and Fink, M.: Therapeutic Studies in Therapy Resistant Schizophrenic Patients, *Compr. Psychiat.*, 7:488–493, 1966.
2. Havens, L. L.: Some Difficulties in Giving Schizophrenic and Borderline Patients Medication, *Psychiatry*, 31:44–50, 1968.
3. Kris, E. B., and Carmichael, D. M.: Follow-up Study on Patients Treated with Thorazine, *Amer. J. Psychiat.*, 112:1022, 1956.
4. Wilcox, D. R. C., Gillan, R., and Hare, E. H.: Do Psychiatric Outpatients Take Their Drugs?, *Brit. Med. J.*, 2:790–792, 1965.
5. Gantz, R. S., and Birkett, D. P.: Phenothiazine Reduction as Cause of Rehospitalization, *Arch. Gen. Psychiat.*, 12:586–588, 1965.
6. Gross, M., et al: Discontinuation of Treatment with Ataractic Drugs, *Recent Advances Biol. Psychiat.*, III, 44–67, 1961.
7. Kris, E. B.: Effects of Pharmacotherapy on Work and Learning Ability: Five Year Follow-up Study, *Recent Advances Biol. Psychiat.*, III, 30–34, 1961.
8. Polvan, N., et al: High and Very High Fluphenazine in the Treatment of Chronic Psychosis, *Proc.*, CINP, 1968. In press.
9. Sanseigne, A. J., et al: New Concept in Phenothiazine Therapy: Fluphenazine Enanthate and Fluphenazine Decanoate, *Agressologie*, 9:3–7, 1968.
10. Barsa, J. A., and Saunders, J. C.: Double-Blind Study of Fluphenazine Enanthate, *Dis. Nerv. Syst.*, 26:496–498, 1965.
11. Bartholomew, A. A., and Holt, N. F.: Long Acting Phenothiazine, Flu-

phenazine Enanthate: Preliminary Communication, *Med. J. Aust.*, 1:12–18, 1966.
12. Blachly, P. H.: Depot Fluphenazine Enanthate Treatment of Outpatient Schizophrenics, *J. New Drugs*, 5:114–116, 1965. ·
13. Kinross-Wright, J., Vogt, A. H., and Charalampous, K. D.: New Method of Drug Therapy, *Amer. J. Psychiat.*, 119:779–780, 1963.
14. Kline, N. S., and Simpson, G. M.: Long Acting Phenothiazine in Office Practice, *Amer. J. Psychiat.*, 120:1012–1014, 1964.
15. Kurland, A. A., et al: Fluphenazine (Prolixin) Enanthate: Phenothiazine Preparation of Prolonged Activity, *Curr. Therap. Res.*, 6:137–147, 1964.
16. Laffan, R. J., High, J. P., and Burke, J. C.: Prolonged Action of Fluphenazine Enanthate in Oil after Depot Injection, *Int. J. Neuropsychiat.*, 1:300–306, 1965.
17. Lambert, P. A., et al: Perspectives nouvelles offertes par un neuroleptique injectable retard l'enanthate de fluphenazine, *Ann. Medicopsychol.*, 124 année, I:702–707, 1966.
18. Pollack, S. L., Tourlentes, T. T., and Zocchi, A. F.: Clinical Trial of Fluphenazine Enanthate: Long Acting Injectable Tranquilizer, *Amer. J. Psychiat.*, 121:73–74, 1964.
19. Ravaris, C. L., Weaver, L. A., and Brooks, G. W.: Controlled Study of Fluphenazine Enanthate in Chronic Schizophrenic Patients, *Dis. Nerv. Syst.*, 26:33–39, 1965.
20. Simpson, G. M., et al: Studies on Second Long Acting Fluphenazine, *Amer. J. Psychiat.*, 121:784–787, 1965.
21. Keskiner, A., et al: Long Acting Phenothiazine (Fluphenazine Decanoate) Treatment of Psychosis, *Arch. Gen. Psychiat.*, 18:477–481, 1968.
22. Itil, T., and Keskiner, A.: Psychopathological and Psychosomatic Rating Scale, Publication 12, St. Louis: Psychiatric Research Foundation of Missouri, 1966.
23. Shapiro, D., and Itil, T.: Cumulative Psychopathological Rating Graph, 1967. In press.
24. Holden, J. M. C., et al: Clinical Laboratory Test Standards in New Drug Trials, *J. Clin. Pharmacol.*, 7:1–8, 1967.
25. Keskiner, A., Holden, J. M. C., and Itil, T.: Maintenance Treatment of Schizophrenic Outpatients With Depot Phenothiazine, *Psychosomatics*, IX:166–171, 1968.
26. Bucci, L., et al: Depot Fluphenazine in Treatment of Psychosis in Community Mental Health Clinic. In press.
27. Keskiner, A., Itil, T., and Holden, J. M. C.: Comparative Study of Fluphenazine Enanthate and Fluphenazine Decanoate in Chronic Schizophrenic Outpatients. In preparation.
28. Gayral, L., and Lambert, P.: "Le Dichlorhydrate de Fluphenazine (Étude des doses élevées et des traitements de longue durée)," in Brill, H., et al (eds.): *Neuropsychopharmacology*, New York: Excerpta Medica Foundation, p. 1128, 1967.

10

*The Therapeutic and Pragmatic Import of Drug Administration Schedules**

by ALBERTO DiMASCIO
and RICHARD D. SHADER

DiMascio and Shader herein make a long-needed contribution to the therapeutic and pragmatic import of drug administration. Basically, they ask the relatively simple question: Why must drugs be given t.i.d. and q.i.d.? They follow with another significant question: May the patient take a drug holiday without its interfering with his progress? Their findings emphasize that conventional drug approaches are too stereotyped and need to be individualized with special drug schedules and holidays. Additionally, the results presented in this chapter will help many of us to observe a reformulation and greater relevancy to drug administration and to render more comfort to the patient while also helping to lower the cost of long-term drug treatment.

It is common and current practice in clinical psychiatry to prescribe psychotropic drugs so that a specified total amount is administered daily in equally divided doses on a three- to six-times-a-day schedule. The rationale for this procedure does not seem to rest on

* Supported in part by NIMH Grant 12279-02.

any scientific basis. Whether it is merely a simple carryover from traditional general medical practice—where drug actions are often short term—or whether it is based on a desire to obtain maximum control of a patient or maximum therapeutic benefit, the practice is inconsistent with what is known about the pharmacology of psychotropic drugs.

Four relevant major facts have been established pertaining to the pharmacological properties of psychotropic drugs:

1. Psychotropic drugs in general have a long biological half-life. For example, a single oral dose of chlordiazepoxide may have a half-life in serum lasting from 8 to 24 hours, and its active metabolites may have a half-life of up to 50 hours.
2. The excretion of psychotropic drugs and their metabolites proceeds at a very slow rate. For example, a single dose of chlorpromazine may be detected biochemically in urine for up to three to four days and behaviorially for 8 to 20 hours.
3. Accumulation of these drugs and their metabolites in various body tissues occurs with continued drug administration, until a saturation level is achieved. On cessation of the drugs, these tissues only very slowly release the accumulations. Traces of the active drug or its metabolites are detectable in urine two to three months later with some drugs.
4. The appearance of the pharmacological properties of these drugs that are of primary clinical value in psychiatry (their antipsychotic or antidepressant effects) is noted later in time (days to weeks) than are the secondary properties (sedation, psychomotor inhibition) or side effects, which are generally most prominently perceived two to six hours after a specific dosage administration.

A consideration of the implications of these factors mitigates against the administration of drugs with the frequency now generally advocated. It is only through a very close scrutiny of these factors and others, such as absorption efficiency, blood and tissue concentrations, and patient body size, that optimal dosage regimens can be *individually* constructed to ensure maximal therapeutic benefit. Such a procedure would be impossible to apply on a widespread basis. However, based on considerations of the above factors, a number of studies have been carried out examining the therapeutic efficacy of a number of different schedules of drug administration. These studies concerned:

1. frequency of daily dosages
2. division of the daily total dosage
3. intermittent drug therapy.

FREQUENCY AND DIVISION OF THE DAILY DOSAGE

In 1958, Tibbits[1] questioned whether the custom of administering chlorpromazine in divided doses was necessary. He explored the feasibility of administering to his patients a single oral dose equal to the total amount they had been receiving in divided doses. Tibbits reported no shift in clinical status or adverse effects other than increased lethargy. His upper range of total dosage, however, was only 200 mg. Haden[2] similarly reported that he found no difference in clinical status of over 400 patients who once had been given their medications (phenothiazines) in divided doses and now were administered the drugs in one large dose at bedtime. Since the drugs were given h.s., the drowsiness they induced became a desirable effect and reduced the need for other hypnotics.

Denber and Travis[3] also examined the frequency of chlorpromazine administration, and concluded that because of side effects noted with a single administration it was necessary to use a twice-daily method; dividing it further proved of no increased benefit. Kramer[4] in 1962 reported a trial of schedule variations in 14 patients on imipramine. He concluded that a single daily dose was as effective clinically as a multiple daily dose schedule. Common side effects were similar, and by specifying the time of day for the single dose, side effects such as dizziness and sedation could be controlled. Peterson and Olson[5] carried out two controlled studies with patients on chlorpromazine or other medications (half the group received their medication h.s. in a single dose, the other half in a multiple dose schedule). A number of rating scales were used to assess clinical status. They reported "not only an absence of negative developments with the once-a-day schedule, but an unanticipated positive effect," such as increased sociability, broadening of interests, and reduction of idiosyncratic behavior. Further, the drug-induced drowsiness was turned to advantage by the h.s. administration. Peterson and Olson limited their patient sample to those who were on 400 mg chlorpromazine (or its equivalent), or less.

Other comparable findings were reported by Roberts,[6] Vestre and

Schiele,[7] Hruska, et al,[8] and Kris,[9] who administered chlorproma-zine (or other phenothiazines) in single doses up to 600 mg (or its equivalent). In an unpublished report emanating from the NIMH Collaborative Study on Chronic Schizophrenia,[10] chlorpromazine was tested in 78 patients at a daily dose of 2,000 mg, administered either in a b.i.d. or a q.i.d. schedule. The former dose was divided so that one third was given in the morning and two thirds in the evening; the latter dose was evenly divided. There was no difference in clinical benefit between the two schedules, though the b.i.d. patients showed fewer side effects. No patient on the b.i.d. schedule was dropped from the study for side effects, though four patients on the q.i.d. schedule had to be terminated. In a study undertaken by the senior author,[11] a b.i.d. schedule was compared with a t.i.d. schedule of drug administration for chlorpromazine or for triflu-operazine in a group of 26 female chronic schizophrenics. With chlorpromazine the ward behavior ratings showed improvement on the b.i.d. schedule after six weeks on the regimen. No other differ-ences—in clinical status ratings or in side effects—were found between the conditions of the two dose schedules for either drug.

Though only a few studies have shown a superiority of the q.i.d. or b.i.d. schedule over the multiple dose schedules, no study has reported the reverse. Other than increased drowsiness, no side effect was observed more often with the q.i.d. or b.i.d. schedule than with the multiple schedules. One note of caution must be mentioned, however; in all the studies cited except the NIMH project, the pa-tients had been on a maintenance dosage or on the medication prior to initiation of the q.i.d. or b.i.d. schedule. Our experience, as well as that of others, suggests that it might be desirable to start an acutely disturbed patient on a multiple dose schedule until some degree of control has been obtained (the mechanism probably being via the sedative-hypnotic and motor-inhibiting properties of the drug rather than through their primary antipsychotic properties), and then switch the patients to the q.i.d. or b.i.d. schedule.

On the q.i.d. schedule, it is suggested that drugs with sedative-hypnotic activity be given near bedtime, to utilize that action of such drugs, as well as make more imperceptible (when patients are asleep) other side effects such as orthostatic hypotension, dry mouth, or visual blurring. Drugs with a tendency to produce stimu-lation or insomnia should be administered early in the morning.

On the b.i.d. schedule, it is suggested that a one third to two thirds division be utilized. For the more sedating type of drugs, the small dose should be given in the morning, the larger dose h.s.; for the more stimulant type of drugs, the larger dose should be given on awakening and the smaller dose in the early afternoon.

INTERMITTENT DRUG THERAPY

In intermittent drug therapy, use is made of the pharmacological facts that there is tissue accumulation of these drugs and their metabolities and that the excretion of these products is very slow. Intermittent therapy may vary from medication every other day or "drug-free" weekends to periodic long-term discontinuations of drugs.

In the DiMascio and Chien study cited above,[11] another phase of the experiment involved omitting on alternate days the administration of any medication; there was no increase in the daily dose to compensate for this omission. Ratings completed at the end of six weeks on this regimen showed a slight deterioration in psychopathology (BPRS scores) but no change in ward behavior ratings or on global mental status assessments. Greenberg and Roth,[12] however, present evidence indicating that chronically ill schizophrenic patients can be maintained on medication administered with a three-times-a-week and even a twice-a-week frequency.

Ayd[13] has extensively reviewed the literature on drug-free holidays, both the short-term (weekends) and the long-term (weeks) discontinuations. The many studies cited[13-20] all support the fact that patients who have been stabilized on a neuroleptic drug will show no clinical deterioration when the drugs are discontinued for two to three days at a time, and the majority of patients can even remain off drugs for up to six months without relapse. It is important to point out that these patients were terminated for experimental purposes and not because they had improved sufficiently to warrant a trial period off drugs. In general, termination of medication was abrupt and not a gradual withdrawal; few ill effects were noted as a consequence of this procedure. The authors cited present data to indicate that 70% to 90% of patients tolerate a no-medication period of one month (ie, show no clinical deterioration), and that 40% to 80% could do so for three to six months. They also show that the substitution of a placebo for the drug when discontinuation is initiated slows down the relapse rate.

Caffey et al[18] also gave an excellent review of the subject and presented data derived from 348 patients from a VA Cooperative

Study. Figure 1 summarizes the findings of the study. They concluded that a no-medication schedule is readily feasible for short periods of time but that for longer lengths (three to four months), though it is still well-tolerated by a small number of patients, many borderline adjustment problems result that would not have been allowed to continue by the staff had the patients not been in a study.

Fig. 1: Cumulative Percentage of Clinical Relapses

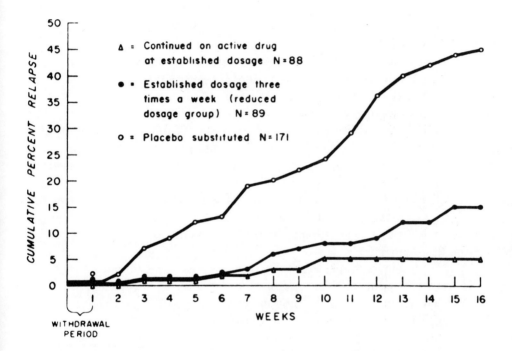

Previously published in *Chronic Diseases;* 17, 347–358, 1964, and reproduced with permission of Pergamon Press, Limited.

SOME THEORETICAL AND PRAGMATIC IMPLICATIONS

The data presented in this chapter clearly demonstrate that a number of revisions can be made in present methods of drug administration *without loss of beneficial effects and in certain instances with greater therapeutic value.*

The use of a q.i.d. or a b.i.d. dose schedule for drug administration, with the suggested timing of the doses, can produce the following beneficial effects:

1. For the patient
   a) less bother from the standpoint of time
   b) fewer tablets to take
   c) fewer and milder side effects during the working hours, thus less discomfort
   d) less need to take antiparkinson drugs, since fewer side effects are perceived
   e) more availability of his own faculties (physical and mental) during the day, since he is not continually sedated
   f) less need to take other hypnotic drugs in the evening
   g) less feeling of complete dependency on drugs
2. For the nursing and medical staff
   a) less time needed to administer drugs
   b) no need to look around for patients during the day to give drugs (Patients can thus be sent out to other therapeutic and recreational activities for almost all day and the staff used for these purposes)
   c) less attention required by patients in regard to their concern and complaints of side effects
   d) less concern about nighttime problems
3. Financially
   a) bigger single doses that are less expensive than an equivalent amount in smaller doses
   b) less need for sleeping medication
   c) less use of antiparkinson drugs
   d) personnel saving in time.

The use of an intermittent drug-therapy schedule can produce the following beneficial effects:

1. For the patient
   a) no need to bother with medications; thus the opportunity to develop the feeling that he is not completely dependent on drugs, which represents to him that he is improving
   b) the opportunity to test out whether he actually needs the medication
   c) the opportunity for the body to rid itself of some of these

       drugs that have accumulated in the tissues and in time show
       up in a variety of body organs (eyes, skin, heart muscles, etc.)
   d) freedom from some of the drugs' side effects that may inter-
       fere with weekend activities

2. For the nursing and medical staff
   a) reduced work load at a time (weekends) when fewer person-
       nel are available; therefore, more time for guidance in recrea-
       tional activities

3. Financial
   a) less or no medication administered
   b) less personnel time needed for this activity.

All these advantages accrue without loss of benefit—and with possible clinical benefit—to the patient. There are those clinicians who maintain that the personal contacts with staff members, brought about through the multiple dosing schedule, are valuable for patients. The overwhelming data do not substantiate this contention, although for specific patients such contacts might play an important role.

No mention has been made in this chapter of the therapeutic and pragmatic impact of long-lasting injectable medications (that would involve a single bimonthly or monthly drug administration sched-ule) because the authors believe sufficient data is not available to make a decisive conclusion. Present evidence, however, suggests that it might be a therapeutically effective method—a method that would elaborate on the pragmatic benefits cited in this article.

REFERENCES

1. Tibbits, J. C. N.: Single Daily Dose of Chlorpromazine, *Lancet*, 1:689, 1958.
2. Haden, P.: Drugs—Single or Multiple Daily Dosage? *Am. J. Psychiat.*, 115: 932–933, 1959.
3. Denber, H. C., and Travis, J. H.: Chlorpromazine in the Treatment of Mental Illness; V: Administrative Problems, *Psychiat. Quart.*, 32:538–544, 1958.
4. Kramer, J. C.: Single Daily Dose Schedules of Imipramine (Tofrānil), *Compr. Psychiat.*, 3: No. 3, 191–192, 1962.
5. Peterson, D. P., and Olson, G. W.: "Single" versus "Multiple"-Dose Ad-ministration of Tranquilizing Medications, Psychiatric Studies and Project No. 14, Washington, D.C., Mental Health Service of the Am. Psychiat. Assoc., pp. 2–4, 1963.
6. Roberts, F. J.: Single Daily Dose Treatment of Psychiatric Patients with Phenothiazine Derivatives, *J. Ment. Sci.*, 107:104–108, 1961.

7. Vestre, M. D., and Schiele, B. C.: An Evaluation of Slow-Release and Regular Thioridazine and Two Medication Schedules, *Curr. Ther. Res.*, 8: No. 12, 585–591, 1966.
8. Hruska, M., Bruck, M., and Hsu, J. J.: Therapeutic Effects of Different Modes of Chlorpromazine Administration, *Dis. Nerv. Syst.*, 27: No. 8, 522–527, 1966.
9. Kris, E. B.: Simplifying Chlorpromazine Maintenance Therapy, *Am. J. Psychiat.*, 114:9, 1958.
10. Prien, R. F.: Personal communication, April 1966.
11. DiMascio, A., and Chien, Ching-piao: Clinical Effects of Various Schedules of Medication: Manuscript submitted.
12. Greenberg, L. M., and Roth, S.: Differential Effects of Abrupt Versus Gradual Withdrawal of Chlorpromazine in Hospitalized Chronic Schizophrenic Patients, *Am. J. Psychiat.*, 123:221–226, 1966.
13. Ayd, F.: Drug Holidays—Intermittent Pharmacotherapy for Psychiatric Patients, *Int. Drug Therapy Newsletter*, 1: No. 8, October 1966.
14. Good, W. W., Sterling, M., and Holtzman, W. H.: Termination of Chlorpromazine with Schizophrenic Patients, *Am. J. Psychiat.*, 115:443, 1958.
15. Olson, G. W., and Peterson, D. B.: Sudden Removal of Tranquilizing Drugs from Chronic Psychiatric Patients, *J. Nerv. Ment. Dis.*, 131:252–255, 1960.
16. Rothstein, C.: An Evaluation of the Effects of Discontinuation of Chlorpromazine, *N. E. J. Med.*, 262:67–69, 1960.
17. Rothstein, C., Zeltzerman, I., and White, H. R.: Discontinuation of Maintenance Dosages, *J. Nerv. Ment. Dis.*, 134:555–560, 1962.
18. Caffey, E. M., Jr., Diamond, L. S., Frank, T. V., Grasberger, J. C., Herman, L., Klett, C. J., and Rothstein, C.: Discontinuation or Reduction of Chemotherapy in Chronic Schizophrenics, *J. Chronic Dis.*, 17:347–358, 1964.
19. Judah, L. N., Josephs, Z. M., and Murphree, O. D.: Results of Simultaneous, Abrupt Withdrawal of Ataraxics in 500 Chronic Psychotic Patients, *Am. J. Psychiat.*, 118:156–158, 1961.
20. Gross, M., and Reeves, W. P.: "Relapses after Withdrawal of Ataractic Drugs: Interim Report (31 patients out of 36) Control Group: 82.1% did not relapse—after 6 months of observation," in Greenblatt, M. (ed.): *Mental Patients in Transition*, Springfield, Ill.: Charles C. Thomas, 1961, pp. 313–321.

TREATMENT
OF AFFECTIVE DISORDERS
IN CLINICAL PRACTICE

11

Treatment of Affective Disorders in Clinical Practice: Implications for Education and Research;* and the Biogenic Amine Hypothesis

by JOHN M. DAVIS

Davis, working for several years at the National Institute of Mental Health, has been reviewing all controlled therapeutic investigations of depressive disorders.† He combines findings of selected studies and treats them statistically. His extensive study shows that monoamine oxidase (MAO) inhibitors give relief to a subtype of patient with depressive disorders; generally, the tricyclic antidepressant drugs relieve the majority of patients. MAO inhibitors are more toxic than the tricyclic antidepressant drugs and less effective. Davis looks with favor on the use of lithium carbonate in the treatment of mania, viewing it as the first psychopharmacologic drug that prevents a syndrome. A large majority of investigators find lithium carbonate to be effective in the treatment of mania, but findings are unclear concerning its help in depression.

---

* Presented in part at the Annual Meeting of the American College of Neuropsychopharmacology, Puerto Rico, December, 1966.

† Space limitations do not permit the listing of the over 700 references reviewed in the preparation of this chapter. A complete bibliography can be obtained by writing the author.

There are many studies that lend hope to the belief that we may be somewhat closer to discovering the chemistry of depression. Davis' summary of investigations being performed that assume a chemical cause of depression opens new doors for future research. His encyclopedic treatment of the subject of depression deserves careful attention, chiefly because of the thoroughness with which he has examined the chemistry and clinical therapy of manic and depressive disorders.

Among the most valuable suggestions offered in this chapter are a new approach in teaching psychopharmacology to psychiatrists and the development of a subdivision of psychopharmacology in the department of psychiatry providing consultation for the other divisions of the hospital.

An extensive number of therapeutic patterns exist in the treatment of manic and depressive disorders. The current clinical approach is to treat the manic or depressed patient with combined or exclusive therapy, dependent on the psychiatrist's convictions. Patients with depressive disorders may be treated with electroconvulsive therapy (ECT), psychopharmacotherapy, or psychotherapy. The drugs in use are tricyclic antidepressants; monoamine oxidase inhibitors (MAO); phenothiazine derivatives: phenothiazines combined with tricyclic antidepressants; MAO inhibitors combined with major or minor tranquilizers; amphetamines, narcotics, or lithium.

The main purpose of this chapter is to make available to the treating psychiatrist data from double-blind, well-designed research studies, in order to present to him possibly better clinical choices in psychopharmacotherapy.

The second purpose is to indicate areas in which definitive research and changes in education are needed to enhance the accuracy of the psychiatrist's clinical judgment and scope.

Tricyclic Antidepressants

Uniformity of clinical opinion concerning the efficacy of the tricyclic antidepressants does not exist. Some psychiatrists report they rarely use ECT, since the majority of their patients respond to tricyclic drugs. A few psychiatrists are uncertain about the efficacy of drug therapy in depression. This opinion seems to be based on several double-blind studies that showed no significant improvement when tricyclic drugs were compared to placebo. From a comparison of 60 investigations relative to tricyclic drugs versus placebo, it is apparent that there is some truth in both beliefs.

Several difficulties obscure definitive results in evaluating the effectiveness of the tricyclic drugs, including the fact that depressive syndromes are a heterogeneous group of disorders, and no specific drug can be expected to benefit every patient.

Many depressed patients improve spontaneously. Klerman and Cole note that 46% of newly hospitalized depressed patients show improvement in the first few weeks of treatment, whereas 16% to 20% of chronic depressions improve during initial treatment. Such spontaneous improvement frequently obscures the drug effect, blurring the outcome of treatment.

Drug efficacies are generally expressed in one of two ways: some investigators enumerate percentages of improved patients treated with drug or placebo; others, using a rating scale, give the mean change in a patient population. Twenty-six of 33 controlled studies comparing imipramine and placebo presented percentage improvement. Combining the data from these 26 studies showed that 734 patients were treated with imipramine and 606 were given placebo. About 70% of the patients treated with imipramine were significantly improved, compared to 39% on placebo. There were no studies in this group where placebo clearly produced greater improvement than imipramine. In subtracting the percentage of improvement with placebo from percentage improvement with imipramine, the average drug-placebo difference was found to be 30.8%. The statistical increment of improvement produced by imipramine is roughly 31% above that produced by placebo. Though this may be considered relatively small, the fact that all studies showed a greater improvement produced by imipramine offers proof that there is only an infinitesimal statistical probability that chance played any part in these results.* The probability of these results,

---

* Several methods exist for combining statistical results from a number of independent studies. Since there are 26 studies that give data on the number of patients improved or not improved with imipramine or with placebo, it is possible in each individual study to compute a chi-square statistic, or another intermediate statistic. Using the two methods discussed by Cochran—one involving a summation of the individual chi-square values divided by the square root of the number of such values, the other involving the computation of a weighted score of proportion improvement with drug and with placebo—an overall statistical statement based on the combined data from all 26 studies can be obtained. Both of Cochran's methods were utilized in the statistical tests computed to combine individual data from all the studies under discussion in this chapter, and thus to arrive at a total statement of statistical probability.

which favor imipramine over placebo, being arrived at by chance was in one instance 10^{-160} and in other instances even less. By increasing sample size, a highly statistically significant result can be obtained proving the drug to be more effective than placebo. It is important to recognize, however, that imipramine is only a moderately effective drug—about 30% of the depressions remained unimproved among the 734 patients.

One may speculate that if it were possible to clearly identify imipramine-responders to obtain a more homogeneous patient sample, a greater therapeutic efficacy could be demonstrated. Dosage schedules may also play a role. Clinical experience indicates that for many of the more severely depressed patients the optimal dosage of imipramine varies from 150 to 250 mg/day. The dosages administered were much less in some of the studies during all or a significant portion of the drug study trial period. Treatment with 75 mg for 15 days, followed by 150 mg for the next seven days, may be an inadequate dosage for many depressed patients.

Jensen and Schulsinger treated 20 patients with intramuscular amitriptyline and compared them to a group receiving the same dosage (75–150 mg) orally. In 50% of the patients in each group it was found that the initial lag period before drug effectiveness occurred was eight days for the group receiving intramuscular amitriptyline, and 16 days for the group receiving oral medication. Alteration of dosage and route of administration, particularly during the initial phase of therapy, might prove useful in attempting to produce a more rapid therapeutic response.

A few patients, most commonly those with schizo-affective disorders, experience an acute exacerbation of psychotic symptoms with tricyclic drugs. This psychotic symptomatology is considered by some to be a superimposed toxic psychosis. Others believe such symptoms to be either the activation of an underlying schizophrenic process or a shift from a depressive to a manic attack. Data collected by Hohn, et al, indicates that the effects of these toxic reactions could cancel out the therapeutic effectiveness of imipramine, thus blurring the pharmacologic effects of this tricyclic drug.

The newer tricyclic drugs are at least as effective as imipramine. Seven double-blind studies with amitriptyline, three with desipramine, and three studies with nortriptyline have shown these drugs to be better than placebo. In addition, two studies with protriptyline, four with opipramol, and one study with trimipramine present evidence that these drugs also are more effective than placebo.

There were a few studies—two with amitriptyline and two with desipramine—that failed to indicate a statistically significant drug effect.

Several double-blind studies show amitriptyline to be superior to imipramine. However, this may be a dosage artifact: comparing these drugs on a milligram to milligram basis, amitriptyline may be slightly more potent. Hordern, et al, in two double-blind studies, found amitriptyline to be slightly superior when both drugs were administered in a schedule of 200 mg/day after the first week. The older, more severely depressed patients also responded better to amitriptyline. Sandifer, et al, administered imipramine and amitriptyline in different dose ratios (maximum dose imipramine, 240 mg/day; amitriptyline, 150 mg/day). Resultant findings indicate that the two drugs were roughly similar in therapeutic efficacy. Two studies show trimipramine to be slightly superior to imipramine. Nevertheless, there is not enough evidence available clearly to show this drug to be more effective than the other tricyclic drugs. Preliminary studies suggest that other tricyclics, such as nortriptyline, protriptyline, desipramine, proheptatriene, and dibenzepin, are roughly equal to imipramine. However, none of the tricyclic drugs has been proved with certainty to be more effective than any other.

Important future research should be directed toward determining whether a given subtype of patient would respond better to one specific tricyclic drug than to another. The agitated depressive might respond better to amitriptyline because of its greater sedative properties, whereas the retarded depressive might respond better to a more stimulating drug such as protriptyline. Amitriptyline is the most sedating drug of the tricyclic group; imipramine, at a similar dosage, is slightly less sedating. The desmethyl derivatives, desipramine and nortriptyline, possess a lesser degree of sedating qualities, the least sedating tricyclic drug is protriptyline. There is no hard and fast evidence that indicates the desmethyl derivatives act appreciably faster than their parent compounds.

Monoamine Oxidase Inhibitors

The monoamine oxidase (MAO) inhibitors comprise the second major class of antidepressant drugs.

Iproniazid was noted to have definite mood-elevating properties when first used in the treatment of tuberculosis. This led to its clinical trial by Crane and later Kline, who found in their preliminary study that iproniazid was an effective antidepressant. Many clinicians who have compared several other MAO inhibitors consider iproniazid to be an outstanding drug in the treatment of depression.

Three of five double-blind studies showed a significantly greater therapeutic improvement with iproniazid when compared to placebo. Of these, one study showed etryptamine to be better than placebo; one study of two demonstrated that pheniprazine was more effective than placebo. Serious toxicity findings, however, have caused all three drugs to be withdrawn from the market in the United States. In two studies, tranylcypromine showed evidence of being effective in the treatment of depression. For a time, this drug also was withdrawn from the United States market because of toxicity. It has been reinstated by the Food and Drug Administration following revised prescription information plus a warning regarding toxicity. Some psychiatrists believe a subtype of patients respond uniquely to tranylcypromine. Pargyline, though found to be slightly inferior to tranylcypromine, offers proof of being an effective antidepressant. Of five studies with isocarboxazid, only one showed the drug to be clearly more effective than placebo. Phenelzine may be an effective MAO inhibitor, but three studies have found nialamide to be ineffective. There is, however, a possibility relative to isocarboxazid and nialamide that the ineffective findings mentioned above may be the result of a dose artifact. Had these drugs been administered in higher doses, perhaps the results might have been different.

Improvement with MAO inhibitors often occurs four to eight weeks after initiation of therapy, its onset frequently being quite dramatic. Since the patients do not generally know when the therapeutic improvement is expected to occur, some investigators have argued that this phenomenon supports evidence for the efficacy of these drugs.

Evidence exists that the antidepressant action of MAO inhibitors is related to their ability to inhibit the enzyme monoamine oxidase. MAO inhibitors may be hydrazines or nonhydrazines. Although these two subclasses differ in many properties, they share one distinctive property—their ability to inhibit monoamine oxidase. Pare, et al, used as subjects terminal patients who had associated depressive states, and demonstrated that the onset of therapeutic effectiveness correlated with the time course of MAO inhibition in the brain.

Consanguine relatives of patients, who also become depressed when treated with tricyclic drugs or MAO inhibitors, will be most likely to respond to the same drug or group of drugs successfully used to treat the patient. Data is needed to validate these interesting observations further.

Patients who do not respond to MAO inhibitors possibly will respond to tricyclic antidepressant drugs; in rare cases, the converse is true. The most effective MAO inhibitors, iproniazid and tranylcypromine, are not completely safe drugs because of their hepatic or vascular toxicity. The tricyclic antidepressants are more acceptable for treatment because of their relative safety and therapeutic effectiveness.

TABLE 1

Effectiveness of Monoamine-Oxidase Inhibitors, Compared to Imipramine, indicating the number of studies in which a Drug was found More, Equally, or Less Effective

Drug	Total No. of Controlled Studies	PERCENTAGE OF STUDIES IN WHICH—		
		Drug was more effective than Imipramine	Drug was equal to Imipramine	Imipramine was more effective
Tranylcypromine	3	—	100%	—
Isocarboxazid	4	—	50%	50%
Pheniprazine	3	—	33%	67%
Phenelzine	7	—	71%	29%
Nialamide	1	—	—	100%

Data comparing tricyclic drugs and MAO inhibitors is summarized in Table 1. MAO inhibitors such as iproniazid and tranylcypromine are about equally effective compared with the tricyclic antidepressants. The other MAO inhibitors—isocarboxazid, pheniprazine, or phenelzine—were found to be less effective than the tricyclic antidepressants.

Amphetamine and Other Psychomotor Stimulants

Psychomotor stimulants such as amphetamine, methylphenidate, deanol, etc., have little effect toward lessening severe depression. They may produce in patients an increased alertness and elation for short periods of time, but their effect is slight and of little clinical value. Side effects of anxiety, tension, and irritability might result from the use of these drugs.

Studies have shown amphetamine to be no better than placebo in treating depressed outpatients. When an amphetamine-chlorpromazine combination was compared to chlorpromazine alone in the treatment of chronic schizophrenics, the chlorpromazine was more effective. In one study, phenelzine proved less effective than placebo in the treatment of depression. In a Veterans Administration Collaborative Study, dextroamphetamine was equal to placebo in treating several hundred neurotic and psychotic depressed patients. Fabing, et al, investigated pipradrol and did not find it an effective antidepressant.

Phenothiazines and Depression

Phenothiazine derivatives have proven to be effective antidepressants. The first placebo-controlled, randomly assigned, double-blind study of phenothiazines was done at Hillside Hospital. This investigation showed that chlorpromazine and imipramine were equally effective, both being superior to placebo in the treatment of agitated depression; only imipramine proved superior to placebo in the treatment of retarded depression. The antidepressant efficacy of chlorpromazine has been verified in an NIMH Collaborative Study. Thioridazine proved to be an effective antidepressant in a VA Collaborative Study. Since many patients who qualify for admission to a Veterans Administration Hospital have had a schizophrenic or schizophrenic-like illness during early adulthood, they may constitute a special population of depressed patients from those in other hospitals. The Veterans Administration has done a series of very closely controlled studies using multivariate analysis. Because the VA population is a relatively homogeneous one, studied with identical or similar rating scales, it is possible to combine results from different VA Hospital studies, as shown on Table 2. There appears to be a small therapeutic efficacy both for phenothiazines and for tricyclic antidepressants. Thioridazine and perphenazine proved to be effective antidepressants in anxious depression. Perhaps the combination of a phenothiazine and an antidepressant drug would be more effective.

There are two aspects of combination therapy to be considered in drug studies. First, it is possible that a single drug may help only a segment of a population. For example, 90% of population A might

TABLE 2

Results of Drug Treatment: Response of VA Patients Classified by Overall-Hollister subtypes. Change measured by IMPS Manifest Depression Score both for subtypes and for the population as a whole (except where noted).

Drug Treatments	OVERALL-HOLLISTER SUBTYPES			Entire Population Change Score
	Anxious	Hostile	Retarded	
Study 1				
Imipramine	38	38	66	43
Thioridazine	64	51	32	56
Study 2				
Amitriptyline	50	52	72	54
Amitriptyline-Perphenazine	66	74	36	64
Study 3				
Tranylcypromine	47	72	15	44
Dextroamphetamine	65	39	38	50
Study 4				
Dextroamphetamine-Amobarbital				34
Placebo				43
Isocarboxazid				27
Imipramine				57
Study 5				
Placebo				45
Desipramine				23
Atropine				39
Imipramine				45
Amitriptyline				54
Study 6				
Amitriptyline	53*	38*	120*	75
Perphenazine	93*	64*	−4*	35
Amitriptyline-Perphenazine	84*	77*	62*	65

* Mean change scores on IMPS total pathology were used, since manifest depression data were not available.

respond to drug alpha and only 10% to drug beta, whereas in population B only 10% might respond to drug alpha and 90% to drug beta. Yet if population A and B consist of equal numbers, a combined score for the entire population would show a 50% average improvement with each drug. This situation is to be differentiated from the one in which a given combination may have a synergistic effect to help a given patient achieve a degree of improvement greater than that with either drug given alone.

It is important in evaluating studies of drug combinations to have control groups for each drug given alone, given in combination, as well as a placebo control group. As observed in Table 2, data on drug combinations in the VA population are presented both in terms of general and specific subtype efficacy.

The perphenazine-amitriptyline combination seems to show particular promise with the hostile type of depression. In several studies based on outpatient populations with anxiety and depression, the amitriptyline-perphenazine combination has proved superior to chlordiazepoxide and placebo. However, the British General Practitioner Research Group, in its study of drug combinations, did not find this combination to be superior to perphenazine alone.

In psychotic depressed and schizo-affective groups, a tranylcypromine-trifluperazine combination was found to be more effective than placebo. This might be a useful combination for certain subtypes of psychotic or severely depressed patients.

Minor Tranquilizers

The therapy of depression in outpatient populations may be somewhat different from that to be observed in more severely ill inpatient populations. In depressions associated with character disorders, Deprol (a combination of meprobamate and benactyzine) and chlordiazepoxide may prove useful. Rickels, et al, compared imipramine and Deprol, finding that the autonomic side effects of imipramine were well tolerated by patients at a university clinic. Sedation was poorly tolerated by this group. Conversely, in a lower-class outpatient population treated in a city hospital, patients were alarmed by autonomic side effects and preferred Deprol, the more sedating compound.

The usefulness of Deprol in outpatients has been confirmed by Gordon, Alvig, and Krebser. In a subsequent study, Rickels, et al, found meprobamate to be an effective medication in the treatment of depression in an outpatient population. However, protriptyline was also an effective antidepressant when its effects were measured after the usual lag period. Outpatients with low anxiety responded particularly well to protriptyline. The combination of meprobamate and protriptyline likewise proved effective.

Though chlordiazepoxide has a euphoric effect, it may be helpful in certain types of chronic depression with character disorders and situational depressions, increasing vigor and energy in some anxious patients. It may reinforce self-assertiveness, aid patients to relate better to their physician, and enable them to view their environment with more optimism. Chlordiazepoxide, diazepam, and oxazepam decrease the possibility of suicide in the depressed patient, since he can ingest large amounts of these drugs without fatal results.

Electroconvulsive Therapy

During the 1940s and 1950s, ECT was the preferred treatment for severe depression. It has continued to be widely used, both in the unmodified form and also modified by the addition of short-acting intravenous barbiturates and muscle relaxants such as succinyl-choline. These modifications do not influence the therapeutic effects, but increase patient acceptance by reducing anxiety and the possibility of fractures. The modifications have failed to diminish cumulative memory disturbances or confusion, and there is the possibility that permanent brain damage may exist.

Unilateral ECT, a recent modification, is claimed in many quarters to be as effective as the conventional techniques with the apparent advantage of producing less impairment of memory and intellectual function. Further research is needed, using tests for right-sided brain damage, to ascertain whether unilateral ECT is as free from brain impairment as is claimed. Nevertheless, there is empiric evidence that conventional ECT does produce a deficit in general and/or left-sided brain functioning, whereas unilateral ECT seems to produce a smaller deficit.

A number of controlled studies have shown ECT to be effective in the treatment of depression, using controls such as seconal groups, no-treatment groups, or placebo. It is difficult to achieve an adequate placebo control for ECT, and barbiturate coma may not mimic the memory deficit resultant from ECT. Placebo groups do provide adequate control for spontaneous improvement. Although there is little doubt of the clinical effectiveness of ECT, a more important issue is the relative effectiveness of ECT when compared with the antidepressant drugs.

Of six studies reviewed comparing ECT and imipramine, two

showed no significant difference between the treatments; three showed ECT to be slightly more effective; one showed that each therapy produced a slightly different pattern of improvement on a wide range of variables.

Greenblatt, et al, found that ECT produced more improvement (89%) than imipramine (73%), phenelzine (83%), or placebo (69%). Isocarboxazid produced less improvement (58%) than imipramine, phenelzine, or placebo. With patients seriously disabled in mood, affect, self-esteem, and cognitive orientation, ECT and imipramine produced more improvement at a faster rate than did isocarboxazid. Those who improved showed a marked lessening in hopelessness, depressed mood, and physical tension, but such items as hostility, guilt, and obsessive thinking remained unchanged. The selectivity of effect may prove of heuristic value in leading to increased investigation of the specificity of antidepressant action.

McDonald, et al, found amitriptyline to be approximately as effective as ECT in the therapy of depressive reactions, with both treatments being more effective than control procedures. ECT proved to be superior to phenelzine in two studies. Other studies showed that after a six-month follow-up iproniazid and ECT were approximately equal in effectiveness, although ECT produced better short-term results.

It is important to note that a number of depressed patients do not respond to treatment with imipramine or phenelzine, whereas approximately 50% of these patients do respond to ECT. Methods should be developed to differentiate patients who would not be helped by imipramine or other antidepressant drugs, but would respond to ECT; such patients should then be started on the treatment of choice without delay.

Mendels studied 105 patients referred for ECT, using a system of weighted variables in an attempt to predict response to ECT. The following negative prognostic factors were isolated: presence of neurotic traits in adulthood, presence of an "inadequate" personality, precipitating factors, hypochondriasis, emotional lability, hysterical attitudes toward illness, the absence of early-morning awakening, previous ECT, good insight, a family history of depression, psychomotor retardation, or delusions. When a sum was obtained from the weighted variables, a low score predicted a good response to ECT. There is a rough similarity between the predictors of response to both ECT and the tricyclic antidepressants.

Many authors agree that mild, long-term depression characterized either by hypochondriasis or, in young people, by episodes of unreality or anxiety fails to respond well to ECT. Results also are poor in chronic depression associated with character disorders accompanied by anhedonia, listlessness, and dejected mood.

The action of ECT may be faster than that of most of the tricyclic antidepressants. This speed factor is an important consideration when treating the acutely suicidal patient.

A review of relapse rates with ECT shows it to vary from approximately 13% to 48% over time periods ranging from six months to three and one half years. The problem of relapse after ECT has been discussed by Hordern, et al. As to the suggestion that maintenance therapy with drugs is necessary to prevent the recurrence of depression after the conclusion of ECT, little evidence exists relevant to measuring the prophylactic effects of long-term imipramine treatment. The mechanism of action of ECT is currently under investigation.

Lithium in Mania and Depression

Lithium, discovered to be effective for mania by Cade in Australia in 1949, was the first effective psychotropic drug of our present psychopharmacologic era. Its discovery constitutes one of the landmarks in psychopharmacology.

Several reasons persist why lithium has not been fully explored and its therapeutic value established: (1) the general commercial and social climate was not prepared in 1949 to exploit a drug so readily and cheaply accessible, nor were there government agencies at that time to support the research of new drugs; (2) at the time Cade published his work the therapeutic climate emphasized psychoanalysis or ECT, and thus was not prepared to accept the significance of this discovery; (3) lithium therapy is associated with potentially toxic hazards, and the drug requires skill in administration. For example, when used in high doses as a salt substitute, lithium proved to be dangerous.

Clinically, lithium is most effective in cases of typical mania, though it also can be effective where there is evidence of delusions and marked irritability. It is believed its effectiveness encompasses all age groups. It is effective in chronic cases, chronic cases with remissions, first attacks, in both sexes; in illnesses of long or short duration. Lithium seems to ameliorate those symptoms most characteristic of mania: manic hyperactivity, irritability, restlessness, and those very typical thought patterns of manic disorders.

The therapeutic range of lithium is fairly specific, seeming to be most effective in manic states. Its action appears to be anti-manic without producing either tranquilization or sedation. The lithium-treated patient is able to feel appropriate happiness, joy, or excitement without manic elation or loss of control.

The qualitative nature of improvement following lithium treatment is superior to that following phenothiazine treatment. After relief, the manic patient appears to approximate his previous personality; he can return to work, and relate to his family at his previous functional level. When given under the careful care of a physician familiar with lithium, there are few toxic side effects. No known toxicity results from long-term administration; there are no acquired tolerance, no addiction, and no withdrawal reactions.

Lithium is inexpensive. Its major disadvantage is that it is a potentially dangerous drug when used in an unsupervised or careless manner. Close supervision is mandatory at all times.

It is important to point out that there are a few cases of manic illness in which lithium has proved ineffectual. Though some of these lithium failures can be attributed to the patient's not taking his prescribed medication, the question arises whether there might be a subtype of mania that is irresponsive, perhaps because of a different etiology than lithium-responsive mania.

The therapeutic effectiveness of lithium in mania is supported by two double-blind studies, a number of clinical investigations in several countries, and by longitudinal data. Schou studied 38 patients divided into "typical" manic cases (N = 30) and "atypical" manic cases (N = 8). The patients were given 900–1800 mg/day of lithium carbonate (some received equivalent doses of other lithium salts). The author's criteria, designed to rule out the possibility of spontaneous improvement, concerned: (1) patients with periodic mania—prevention of the recurrence of manic attacks; (2) constantly manic patients—a decrease in the degree of mania during lithium administration and an increase during placebo substitution; (3) patients with mania rapidly changing in intensity—significantly longer neutral periods during lithium therapy; and (4) significant shortening in the length of the manic phase in patients with previous periodic mania attacks. A total of 14 patients met these criteria; 18 patients showed improvement but did not meet the criteria; and no response was observed in six patients. The combined improvement rate for "typical" manic cases (90%) was higher than that for the "atypical" group (62%).

Maggs conducted a randomly assigned, double-blind, crossover evaluation of patients given lithium or placebo for the first two weeks of the study, followed by a two-week period of no therapy, plus a final two-week period on the alternate therapy, lithium or placebo. Significant improvement occurred with lithium compared to placebo. In longitudinal studies of a few patients with a placebo control, it was demonstrated that during the acute phase of the manic illness, patients would relapse within several days of discontinuation of lithium and substitution of placebo.

A summary of the clinical studies with lithium is given in Tables 3 and 4. Though the general method of study has been the natural history approach, replication of these successes is high. The successful treatment of manic patients with lithium in a variety of settings, in many different countries, confirms the probability of its usefulness. There is but one adverse study, the results of which were based on only two manic patients, who were not helped.

Long-term lithium maintenance also has been found independently by Schou et al, Hartigan, and Baastrup to have an effective

TABLE 3

The Treatment of Mania with Lithium: Studies Listing Marked, Some, or No Improvement

	NUMBER OF PATIENTS IN WHICH THERE WAS		
Authors	Marked Improvement	Some Improvement	No Change
Schlagenhauf (1966)	10	0	0
Rice (1956)	14	20	3
Glesinger (1954)	5	10	6
Kingstone (1960)	11	5	1
Schou, et al (1954)	14	18	6
Wharton (1966)	11	6	8
Warwick (1966)	1	0	0
Williamson (1966)	3	0	0
Hartigan (1963)	17	9	11
Teulie, et al (1955)	16	4	5
Gershon and Yuwiler (1960)	2	0	0
Total	104	72	40

TABLE 4

**The Treatment of Mania with Lithium: Studies Listing
Only Improvement or No Improvement**

Authors	NUMBER OF PATIENTS IN WHICH THERE WAS	
	Improvement	No Improvement
Jacobson (1965)	16	1
Baastrup (1964)	11	0
Cade (1949)	10	0
Despinoy and DeRomeuf (1951)	3	0
Reyss-Brion and Grambert (1951)	3	1
Deschamps and Denis (1952)	4	0
Duc and Maurel (1953)	3	1
Giustino (1953)	0	2
Sivadon and Chanoit (1955)	10	0
Gershon and Trautner (1956)	9	1
Andreani, et al (1958)	13	1
Belling (1959)	24	8
Schou (1959)	91	28
Ashburner (1950)	12	0
Noack and Trautner (1951)	29	1
Total	238	44

prophylactic effect against manic-depressive relapses. The use of medication to prevent an attack of a severe mental disease has constituted an enormous advance in preventive psychiatry. In this advance, no other drug within the scope of our knowledge has as definitive a prophylactic effect as lithium. Its help in preventing severe recurrent conditions, many of which result in suicide or chronic disability, is an outstanding contribution to patient and doctor alike.

In a longitudinal study on the prophylactic use of lithium by Baastrup, 88 manic-depressive females experienced relapses occurring an average of one every eight months prior to lithium therapy. After lithium therapy, relapse frequency dropped to one every 60 months. When lithium was discontinued, relapses occurred in 22 of 25 of these patients, usually within three to four months. Many of these relapses were traceable to inadequate doses of the drug. It is also noteworthy that one third of the relapses occurred during the first six months of therapy, thus suggesting that length of the symptom-free period and experience with adequate control very possibly plays a role in successful prophylaxis. Long-term lithium therapy did not impair mental status or interfere with the normal range of emotion, and no long-term toxic effects have as yet been noted. If Baastrup's work were further substantiated it would have important implications, since the use of prophylactic lithium conceivably could revolutionize the treatment of manic-depressive disorders.

Dosage in the acute treatment phase is usually three to eight 300-mg tablets of lithium carbonate per day, depending on the age, size, health, and psychiatric condition of the patient. Slightly lower doses are indicated for elderly patients. Lithium blood levels should be in the range of 1.2 to 1.6 mEq/L. For the determinations, blood is drawn in the morning prior to any medications. Since this dose level is close to the renal capacity for excretion of lithium, particular care should be taken after seven to ten days to monitor blood lithium levels and, most importantly, side effects. In many cases a steady level of lithium in the blood can be achieved by appropriate fixed dosage schedules, although there is some variation between the absolute dose administered and the serum level observed. In rare cases (less than 1%), lithium accumulates and blood levels are rapidly elevated to toxic levels; medication must then be discontinued immediately.

After control of acute mania, or when given for prophylactic purposes, lithium should be administered in doses sufficient to achieve maintenance blood levels of approximately 0.6 to 0.9 mEq/L.

In research studies and in certain clinical situations it is important to give lithium alone. Since there is a lag period in some patients of 6 to 20 days before the therapeutic effect takes place, it may be advisable to administer a phenothiazine or haloperidol so that the patient can achieve quicker control of his manic symptoms. Such combinations have been used extensively. There are no special hazards attached to their use, and they result in a considerable short-term yet important clinical gain.

Although studying blood levels is helpful in the management of the acute phase of mania, the most important requirement for safety is a good doctor-patient and doctor-family relationship so that the doctor will be notified whenever the patient experiences any symptom that could indicate lithium toxicity. The details of practical management of patients with lithium—the side effects of lithium and their significance—have been reviewed elsewhere.

In the main, lithium has not been found to be effective in most cases of depression, although it is helpful in a few cases. It is difficult to rule out spontaneous remission in improved cases. Nevertheless, the possibility does exist that a small subgroup of depressed patients would respond to lithium.

In summary, it may be concluded from the studies described in this chapter that those psychiatrists who have carefully investigated lithium consider it to have a great degree of clinical efficacy for the treatment of mania. Quantitative research should be done to increase the validity of these findings, as well as to assess its role as a prophylactic drug for mania and depressive disease.

Future Directions and Conclusions

The present, changing therapeutic patterns for effective treatment have been reviewed. The decision to use one treatment or a combination of treatments must remain based on clinical convictions. We have not tried to identify clearly a subgroup of patients who respond uniquely to a specific treatment. Somatic therapy of affective disorders helps a significant majority of patients. This offers the possibility of isolating etiologic factors and leads to the formulation of the biogenic amine hypothesis.

Research to evaluate the effectiveness of antidepressants, as well as to develop new drugs for depression, requires wide knowledge and experience with pharmacology. If amines are involved in depression, either in an etiologic or in a secondary role, knowledge of the biochemistry and pharmacology of amines is important toward psychiatric investigation. Currently, a scientific multidisciplinary psychiatry is evolving. Changes are occurring similar to those that have taken place in the other medical specialties. The research internist, for example, is often both clinician and scientist.

A decade ago, psychiatrists were characterized by Redlich and Hollingshead as being directive-organic or psychoanalytic. Today's subspecialties in psychiatry are special cases in point: the community psychiatrist must deal with the complicated interaction of social factors as they exist in the community; the social research psychiatrist depends on the basic behavioral sciences—psychology, sociology, anthropology, political science, and urbanology; the research psychiatrist specializing in psychosomatic medicine needs special knowledge of internal medicine, anatomy, physiology, and biochemistry. The psychiatrist interested in psychologic processes must have a background in academic psychology dealing with child, abnormal, and personality theory. Psychiatrists interested in aspects of psychoses and their neuropsychopharmacologic treatment must be trained in the psychologic, biochemic, and pharmacologic basic sciences.

The development of these new subspecialties in psychiatry presents new challenges to psychiatric education. Traditionally, psychotherapy was the paradigm for most of the resident's education, and psychodynamic interpretation done under *individual supervision* was the principal approach. Teaching must now be broadened for the residency to meet all the new exploding changes. The paradigm of psychotherapy is not adequate in all respects for the subspecialties. Psychopharmacology is a case in point. Many psychiatric residency programs in psychopharmacology are superficial and informal, with insufficient didactic teaching, formal supervision, or clinical practice.

Revised models of training are needed so that psychiatrists can utilize the multidisciplinary approaches related to the changing patterns of psychiatric care. Certainly, formal didactic training in the principles of basic pharmacology is an important aspect of residency groundwork. In addition, drug rounds and drug consultations under supervision should be considered important additional training. The medical model is helpful where consultants in the subspecialties of medicine are used to help train interns and residents—ie, a consultation with a cardiologist for patients with heart problems, and with an endocrinologist for patients within that subspecialty of problem.

Consultations often are performed by relatively senior residents under the supervision of a faculty member working in that subspecialty. Such teaching is valued by the house staff. What is less frequently discussed is the educational value of the subspecialist to the senior faculty members. For example, the endocrinologist, busy with basic research, may have only a small private practice; thus, the opportunity for him to see great numbers of interesting patients with endocrine problems, through the hospital's consultation process, increases the scope of his experience.

It would seem reasonable, in academic departments of psychiatry, to have some members of a given department who are familiar with psychopharmacology, and who would be able to contribute their special skills to the care of patients and the training of residents, to act in the same manner as does the internal medicine subspecialist. Such a procedure would provide opportunities to acquire much more skill in psychopharmacology. If a member of the department of psychiatry trained in psychopharmacology were responsible, not only for consulting with the house staff of his own department but also for consulting with other medical specialists, an important hiatus that presently exists in current training would be bridged. This psychiatric specialist would train residents in the principles of basic biochemistry and pharmacology with didactic lectures; he would individually supervise drug rounds and drug consultations, individually supervise residents, and act as a catalyst to explore new and more effective teaching methods.

In sum, the newer effective psychopharmacologic agents for the treatment of affective disorders raise new challenges requiring more definitive research. Many important problems in research remain only partially solved. More effective and faster-acting drugs are needed. The subtypes of affective disorders must be more clearly identified so that it can be determined in advance which single or combined drug to use in psychopharmacotherapy. There is a large group of patients who are not responsive to any form of treatment. The ultimate prevention of relapses and suicides remains a problem to be solved. Psychotherapy is undoubtedly extremely important, but more knowledge of the psychology of depression and its psychotherapy is needed. There may be some clues to the etiologic factors in depression, though present evidence is incomplete and inconclusive.

We have described the majority of the effective forms of treatment of affective disorders. Our main challenge is to evolve better psychiatric teaching programs so that we can make all psychiatrists aware of the changing patterns of psychiatric care and the need for improving their skills as clinicians, scientists, and educators.

THE BIOGENIC AMINE HYPOTHESIS

Although definitive knowledge of the causative biochemical factors of depression is lacking, there is clinical evidence that depressions do respond to treatments such as ECT, tricyclic drugs, and MAO inhibitors—all of which have similar or related biologic mechanisms of action. Since reserpine and the MAO inhibitors have shown effects on mood and on norepinephrine (NE) or serotonin (5-HT), beginning in the late 1950s Everett and Toman, Pare and Sandler, and Rosenblatt, et al, postulated that changes in brain NE or 5-HT may be related in depression. Pare and Sandler, in line with these observations, treated depressions with dihydroxyphenylalanine (DOPA), a precursor of NE, and with 5-hydroxytryptophan (5-HTP).

The biochemistry of these drugs, which cause or benefit depression, does lead to testable hypotheses about the etiology of depression and mania, and should generate further research. In this review an interdisciplinary approach will be utilized, a paradigm that involves biology, biochemistry, neuropharmacology, psychopharmacology, and clinical psychiatry. The biology of biogenic amines, as well as some of the more significant evidence relevant to the biogenic amine hypothesis of mania and depression, will be briefly reviewed, and the relationship of different treatments to this hypothesis will be discussed.

TABLE 5

Outline of Factors in the Catecholamine Hypothesis, Showing Postulated Effects of Various Drugs and Antidepressant Therapies on Brain NE and Serotonin Levels

Drug or Treatment	Effect in Man	Effects on Brain Amines
Imipramine and other tricyclic drugs	Benefit depression	Competitively inhibit re-uptake of released amines such as serotonin and NE; thus increase brain levels of serotonin and NE
Monoamine oxidase inhibitors	Benefit depression	Block breakdown of NE and serotonin; thus increase brain levels of NE and serotonin
Electroconvulsive therapy	Benefits depression	Increases turnover and utilization of NE
Lithium	Benefits mania	Increases net uptake of NE; increases levels of deaminated NE metabolites
Reserpine	Causes depression in some patients	Interferes with storage of NE and serotonin in synaptic vesicles; decreases brain levels of NE and serotonin
Alpha-methyl dopa	Causes depression in some patients	Displaces NE from the neuron; thus may lower brain levels of NE

Note that Table 5 is an outline of the biogenic amine hypothesis. Reserpine and similar drugs lower brain levels of 5-HT and NE, thus causing depression. The MAO inhibitors and the tricyclic antidepressants may make more NE or 5-HT available at the receptor site and thus benefit depression. ECT increases NE synthesis and utilization. Lithium may increase the net retention or accumulation of NE or 5-HT. The evidence most relevant to each aspect of the catecholamine hypothesis will be discussed, including evidence supplied by studies of reserpine, MAO inhibitors, tricyclic antidepressants, ECT, lithium, and amphetamine.

NE is a catecholamine located in the peripheral sympathetic fibers, where it functions as a neurotransmitter; it is also concentrated in specific structures in the brain, where it probably functions as a neurotransmitter or as a neuromodulator. NE is stored in intracellular synaptic vesicles, and is present in body fluids and in cell sap. It is continuously being synthesized, broken down, and released. Specifically, the stages of NE synthesis involve the conversion of the amino acid tyrosine to 3, 4-dihydroxyphenylalanine (DOPA), which is converted to dihydroxyphenylethylamine (DOPAMINE), which, in turn, is hydroxylated to NE in the synaptic vesicles. The first stage of synthesis—the tyrosine to DOPA stage—is the rate-limiting stage of the synthesis.

NE is broken down through two pathways: (1) MAO metabolizes NE inside the cell to form 3, 4-hydroxymandelic acid (DHMA), which is then O-methylated by the enzyme catechol-O-methyl-transferase (COMT) to 3-methoxy-4-hydroxy mandelic acid (VMA). (2) Circulating and released NE is initially methylated by COMT to normetanephrine, following which it may be conjugated or deaminated by MAO. Normetanephrine and DHMA may also be further metabolized to 3-methoxy-4-hydroxy phenylglycol (MHPG) and excreted as $MHPG-SO_4$. Thus, the major metabolites of NE excreted in urine are VMA, normetanephrine, and MHPG.

NE or 5-HT is conserved by a process in which nerves take up released NE so that it can be stored and reused. In addition, the actions of these amines are terminated by their re-uptake. 5-HT is localized in the brain, in areas concerned with emotions and sleep; 5-HT may also act either as a neurotransmitter or neuromodulator. It is synthesized from tryptophan by hydroxylation to 5-hydroxytryptophan, which is then decarboxylated to form serotonin (5-HT). 5-HT is metabolized to 5-hydroxyindoleacetic acid.

Reserpine Depression

A significant percentage of hypertensive patients treated with high doses of reserpine develop depression. Reserpine-induced depressions are similar in many respects to endogenous depressive reactions. We have recently reviewed the treatment of patients with reserpine and documented 187 cases of reserpine-induced depression. In some studies the incidence of these depressions was as high as 15%. Hypertensive patients treated with reserpine showed significantly more depressive reactions than similar patients who were treated with other antihypertensive drugs. One third of the reserpine-depressed patients required hospitalization, 19 improving shortly after the drugs were stopped; five required ECT. Most cases of induced depression occurred in patients receiving 0.75 mg/day or more of reserpine. In a study by Lemieux, et al, it was found that reserpine-induced depressions occurred in 30/195 cases (15%), whereas no cases of depression were observed in patients treated with other antihypertensive drugs.

The onset of depression occurs between one and seven months after treatment has begun; however, it has occurred as early as one week and as late as 14 months after initiation of treatment. The evidence for reserpine-induced depression is reinforced by the fact that there is improvement when the patient is taken off reserpine, and depression recurs when the drug is restarted. Another drug similar to reserpine in reducing brain NE and 5-HT is tetrabenazine, reported to be associated with depression. It can be stated that a greater incidence of depression is experienced in those patients treated with reserpine than with other antihypertensive drugs. In addition, the higher the dose of reserpine, the more likely it becomes that the patient will develop a depression.

Reserpine depletes the brain of 5-HT and NE. Evidence from a variety of sources suggests that reserpine disrupts the storage process by which the vesicles store NE, releasing NE into the cell sap, where it is destroyed by mitochondrial monoamine oxidase, hence inactivated intracellularly without exerting any physiologic effect. In animals, reserpine produces a syndrome of sedation, which has been suggested by Brodie, Sulser, and their collaborators to be analogous to depression in man. The sedative effect is correlated, not with total brain amine levels, but rather with the lack of the capacity of the brain to accumulate amines.

When the enzymatic hydroxylation of tryptophan is inhibited by para-chloro-phenylalanine, the levels of 5-HT in the brain are reduced to less than 10% of normal, without marked changes in NE content. Sedation has not generally been observed under these conditions; however, when reserpine is added, and the brain further depleted of 5-HT, animals become sedated. If the animals are specifically depleted of NE by the use of a synthesis inhibitor, alpha-methyl-para-tyrosine, sedation is observed. It must be stressed that any single interpretation of evidence in such a complicated field as catecholamine and 5-HT metabolism must be viewed with caution. In this regard, other interpretations of reserpine sedation should be studied.

The reserpine model of depression has been used as a screening test for antidepressant agents. Pretreatment with either MAO inhibitors or imipramine-type drugs will convert reserpine sedation into an excited state. It has been observed that, using alpha-methyl-para-tyrosine treatment, NE is necessary for excitation to occur. After pretreatment with desmethylimipramine, the deamination of NE released by reserpine treatment is decreased, and the amount of NE and normetanephrine is relatively increased. Reserpine sedation and reserpine model depression can be reversed in animals by DOPA. It has been shown by Degwitz, et al, that patients treated with reserpine become tired and lethargic; this feeling of tiredness or lethergy can be reversed for several hours by treatment with L-DOPA. It is also relevant to note that reserpine administered after unsuccessful treatment with imipramine has produced improvement.

The drug alpha-methyl-dopa has been used to treat hypertension in man. It depletes the brain of norepinephrine through a quite different mechanism than reserpine, involving false transmitters that displace NE from the nerve endings. Alpha-methyl-dopa has been noted to cause depression in a few patients. These depressions can occur fairly rapidly after initiation of treatment with alpha-methyl-dopa.

Antidepressants, MAO Inhibitors, and Tricyclic Drugs

The MAO inhibitors presumably act by blocking the intracellular breakdown of NE and 5-HT by monamine oxidase. This may lead to accumulation of higher levels of the amines in the cell sap.

The potentiation of the action of NE by imipramine and similar drugs in a variety of systems has been explained by the observation that imipramine blocks the uptake of NE or 5-HT into the nerve ending, hence leaving just released NE or 5-HT at the receptor site for a longer period of time. The rate of change of NE at the receptor site could be important.

It should be noted that tricyclic drugs increase the urinary excretion of O-methylated amines and decrease 5-HT uptake in platelets drawn from patients under treatment with imipramine, in comparison to platelets drawn from controlled, drug-free patients. Thus, there is evidence from studies on human depressed patients that the tricyclic drug dose given functions in the manner expected from animal studies.

A similar mechanism exists for neuronal uptake of 5-HT. Using a preparation of broken-off nerve endings, Colburn and the author have demonstrated that nerve endings from rat brain concentrate NE against a concentration gradient, a process that is essentially the re-uptake mechanism. Similar work in brain slices has also demonstrated that brain tissues can take up 5-HT in a manner similar to NE. Using the analogy of the transport carrier system to enzymatic kinetics, Colburn and the author studied the net uptake of NE, 5-HT, and metaraminol into brain nerve-ending particles using different substrates. It is of interest that the inhibition by the tricyclic drugs was found to be competitive. The finding in a therapeutic trial by Prange, et al, following a clinical observation by Kane, that triiodothyronine hastens recovery with imipramine may prove to be both of practical importance and a clue for further research. Also important are the observations that pretreatment with dexamethasone may speed up response to imipramine, as well as the observation by Kurland, and Cumming and Kort, who noted that prednisone or hydrocortisone may help alleviate depression.

Electroconvulsive Shock

Injecting radioactively labeled norepinephrine intracisternally prior to electric shock, Schildkraut, et al, observed that levels of labeled NE in the brain are decreased in shocked animals relative to controls; however, normetanephrine levels are increased. These findings suggest that the rate of neuronal discharge of NE in the brain may be increased by electric shock. Kety, et al, using a technique based on measurement of specific activity of labeled amines 24 hours after a series of electroshock treatments, found a more rapid fall of specific activity in shocked animals than in control animals. This suggests that, following shock, there is an increase in the synthesis and utilization of NE.

Lithium

Schildkraut, et al, found that lithium administered to animals prior to injection of intracisternal NE decreased the levels of labeled normetanephrine and increased the levels of tritiated deaminated catechol metabolites in the brain. Colburn and the author have isolated broken-off nerve endings from brains of animals pretreated with lithium, and compared these to brains of control animals. Initially, it was found that lithium pretreatment increased the net uptake of NE into brain. In a subsequent experiment, it was demonstrated that in a sodium-potassium-magnesium-buffered system there is a small increase in net uptake of NE, metaraminol, and 5-HT. The increased net uptake of NE seen in lithium-pretreated tissue is present in nerve-ending particles that also have been treated with reserpine. Even though reserpine reduced the total synaptosomal accumulation of NE, the increased accumulation in the lithium-pretreated synaptosomes is present at all concentrations of reserpine. Lithium salts also increase the turnover of biogenic amines in the brain. It is noteworthy that the biogenic studies of the interaction of lithium with amines were undertaken as a sole result of the clinical effects of lithium on mania.

Amphetamine

Acute administration of amphetamine causes elation in humans and hyperactivity in animals. This reaction in animal studies has been shown to depend on the presence of catecholamines in the brain.

Tachyphylaxis occurs clinically with amphetamine, which may explain why amphetamine is not an effective antidepressant in humans. It should also be remembered that amphetamine in large doses depletes the brain of NE; prolonged use of this drug is sometimes followed by depression and fatigue. The action of amphetamine on a pharmacologic level is quite complex, and the drug may, in fact, have a number of mechanisms of action. It has been known to decrease rebinding of catecholamines, release catecholamines, possibly have a direct action on the receptor site, and act as an inhibitor of monoamine oxidase in certain situations.

Human Studies

Since 5-HT and norepinephrine do not pass the blood-brain barrier, it is difficult to do meaningful studies using peripheral metabolites or amines. Urinary levels primarily reflect synthesis as well as metabolism in the periphery. It is quite possible that if there is an abnormality of biogenic amine function, it could exist both in peripheral systems and central systems. A number of authors have, therefore, studied various indexes of peripheral amine function. A few of the more pertinent studies relevant to this type of research follow.

Rodnight found that the urinary excretion of tryptamine was significantly decreased in patients suffering from depression, in comparison to normal controls or schizophrenic patients. Coppen and his collaborators found a decreased excretion of urinary tryptamine during depression, in comparison to that observed after recovery. In addition, following a large tryptophan load (50 mg/kg body weight), it was observed that the excretion contained lower amounts of tryptamine during depression than after recovery. These interpretations were based on the hypothesis that urinary tryptamine is produced by decarboxylation of tryptophan in the kidney. These same investigators (Coppen, et al) intravenously injected C^{14} 5-hydroxytryptophan, and measured the rate of expiration of radioactive carbon dioxide. In initial studies, it seemed that the rate of decarboxylation was slowed in depression; subsequent studies have shown no consistent trend.

There have been a number of studies of the endogenous excretion of NE and its metabolites in depressive and manic conditions. Though some depressed patients excrete large amounts of NE and VMA during a psychotic episode, the significance of urinary studies is problematic. Studies related to this significance have been reviewed elsewhere. Rosenblatt and Chanley infused radioactive-labeled norepinephrine into a group of depressed patients and, in contrast to neurotic depressions or other control patients, observed an increase in the ratio of amines to deaminated metabolites in those patients classified as manic-depressive.

Prange, et al, reported that the blood pressure response to infused NE is enhanced in patients after their recovery from depression, as compared to measurements taken during their pretreatment phase of maximal illness.

Since it has been postulated that depression is associated with low

NE brain levels, and since it has been suggested that significant quantities of brain catecholamines are metabolized to 3-methoxy-4-hydroxy-phenylglycol (MHPG), the amount of MHPG excreted in the urine may reflect the metabolism of NE in the brain. In a pilot study, urinary levels of MHPG were found to be significantly lower in a group of seriously depressed patients than in controls.

Because of the difficulty in interpreting urinary amine studies, since amines do not pass out of the brain, investigators have looked for evidence in brain tissue and in the cerebrospinal fluid, hoping that such evidence may more directly reflect the function of brain amines. Two different groups have shown that depressed patients have decreased levels of 5-hydroxy indoles, presumably 5-hydroxy-indole acetic acid, in comparison to controls. These determinations were made on a relatively small number of patients, and further research is necessary to help toward a decision whether CSF-5-hydroxy-indole acetic acid reflects primarily brain concentration indoles. Even if so, other factors such as the concentration gradient of 5-hydroxy-indole acetic acid within the CSF system, the effects of exercise, age, etc., need to be investigated.

Suicide brains were found to have lower 5-HT than controls in an initial study by Shaw, et al. In a subsequent study performed by this author, et al, suicide brains were found to have lower 5-HIAA levels than controls. In summarizing these studies, some of which are obviously limited, we find that a great deal of indirect evidence is consistent with the biogenic amine hypothesis, but the etiology of depression remains unknown.

Several attempts have been made to use the catecholamine and serotonin hypothesis to predict potential treatments for depression, such research also serving as a test of the hypothesis. If there is a deficit of norepinephrine in the brain of depressed patients, it can be predicted that if levels of NE in the brain could be increased, depression could benefit. Much the same reasoning might be applied to 5-HT. One cannot increase norepinephrine in the brain by giving peripheral norepinephrine or DOPAMINE, since these compounds do not pass the blood-brain barrier. DOPA does pass the blood-brain barrier, at least to some extent in specific doses. Pare and Sandler, Turner and Merlis, and Klerman et al have given DOPA to patients; the author has also treated 24 depressed patients with DOPA. Although behavioral changes have been observed, it is quite clear that DOPA has not produced significant improvement in depressed patients in these studies. Coppen et al, as well as Pare, has demonstrated that tryptophan, given in combination with a MAO inhibitor, can hasten the rate of improvement as compared to patients given MAO inhibitors alone. Furthermore, tryptophan, when given alone, can produce improvement in depressed patients. Drugs that block receptors also can provide information. Methysergide, a serotonin antagonist, may be of benefit in mania.

All these experiments and their results are suggestive, and comprise an invitation for future research using what has been done as guidelines. We are far removed from a complete understanding of the etiology of depression. There is evidence, however, that points toward a probable relationship between the biogenic amines and depression.

It is hoped that the review of evidence presented here related to the biogenic amine hypothesis will stimulate others to carry the torch forward.

NEW APPROACHES

TO RESEARCH

AND EDUCATION

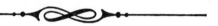

12

The Importance of Diagnosis:
An Analysis and Program[1]

by DONALD F. KLEIN

E. Georget (1795–1828) *wrote his thesis called dissertation* Sur le Causes de la Folie (1820) *for Esquirol, followed by his masterpiece,* De la Folie, *published the same year. In these volumes he was the first to describe a unitary concept of psychopathology. Georget believed that mental illness was a brain disease; his clinical descriptions, though ingenious and thorough, were based on the theory that mental illness was organic. Freud, in 1914, said: "We must bear in mind that all our psychological ideas are, as it were, provisional—psychologische vor laufigkeiten—and will have therefore at some future time to be based on an organic foundation."*

In a study done by Zigler and Phillips among a group of psychologists and psychiatrists, it was discovered that American psychiatrists of the 20th century, in general, believed the cause of mental illness to be psychological whereas European psychiatrists believed it to be organic. This finding evidences the unconscious social and political beliefs of each group. Zigler and Phillips also believe in a unitary concept of psychopathology, their belief being based on psychologic, cultural, and social relationships. They view the relationship between diagnoses and symptomatology as being so slight that to label mental disorders as specific diseases is inaccurate. Later, they contended that as long as diagnosis is confined to the broadest diagnostic categories it is reasonably reliable, but the reliability diminishes as one proceeds from broad inclusive class categories to more narrow and specific ones.

Zigler and Phillips further believe that rather than judge psychiatric

[1] Adapted in part from *Diagnosis and Drug Treatment of Psychiatric Disorders,* and reprinted with permission of Williams and Wilkins, Baltimore, Maryland.

symptoms as expressions of diseases, we can see them simply as a person's behavior as he tries ineffectually to cope with the problems that are unique in his life and beyond his capabilities to master. They dismiss the significance of the biologic base of mental illness, and report only syndromes that are indicative of the person's reaction to his environment, culture, and historic period.

The following two chapters by Rosen, Klein, and their colleagues on social competence show that different diagnostic categories give different results, thereby weakening the significance of the Zigler-Phillips' findings and, in essence, invalidating the only measurable factor supporting the unitary concept of psychopathology. Furthermore, Klein, in his studies on diagnosis and drugs in psychiatry, demonstrates a significant correlation between the two variables. He believes that psychopathology is associated with an intermingling of social, biologic, and psychologic variables. Klein shows the importance of a multidisciplinary approach to schizophrenia, which clearly covers a multifactorial theory of psychopathology.

A major difficulty in outlining the differential indications for psychiatric treatment is the sadly confused state of psychiatric diagnosis. The field is polarized between the unitary theorists who claim that there is no (or at most one) mental illness, and those who believe that every discernible group of symptoms represents a separate and discrete illness with a separate and discrete cause.

Criticisms of the existence or utility of discrete diagnostic entities derive from the unitary approach. However, considerable theoretical disunity exists within this camp.

Karl Menninger, in his scholarly review,[2] has attributed classification to an economizing principle of the human intellect. Though this sounds reasonable, such a formulation obscures whether there are real discontinuities between psychiatric patients. Menninger states: "The unitary concept does not dispense with the descriptive designations. These we must have if they can be cast in a form that will not deny the essential unity of the process." Further: "We propose to think of all mental illness as being essentially the same in quality and differing quantitatively."

Menninger defines mental illness as a variable, hierarchical defensive response to stress; therefore, his theory is not etiologically unitary. Menninger's work respects the range of phenomenologic reality, and he emphasizes meticulous patient study as necessary for a planned ameliorative intervention. Unfortunately, his therapeutic optimism results in prognostic nihilism.

These values are lost by Thomas Szasz's unitary theory, which holds that there is no such thing as mental illness at all, only varieties of gamesmanship.[3] This theory is doubly unitary, since there are no illnesses and only one treatment.

In an attempt to develop prognostic efficiency, Zigler and Phillips[4] have promulgated yet another unitary theory. They postulate an underlying prognostic sociopsychologic dimension, social competence, that cuts across all mental illness. This formulation has the sterling merit of being testable, and as we have shown[5] does not withstand validation.

All such theories reflect an impatience with pettifogging categoric distinctions of no practical or theoretic import. Unfortunately, such unitary theories also inhibit the development of a systematic descriptive classification with demonstrable treatment and prognostic value.

In sharp contrast to unitary approaches, medicine has historically advanced through discovery of disease entities that have corresponding qualitative typologic regularities associated with them. Therefore it is not surprising that such a traditional diagnostic approach should be part of medical psychiatric ideology. On the other hand, the history of applied psychology has consisted of the determination of certain measures, such as IQ, which then have been quantitatively related to validity criteria, such as school achievement. This tradition has resulted in the belief by many psychologists that categories and diagnostic types are simply crude approximations of the underlying reality, useful only as terminologic conveniences. That is, for many purposes it is adequate to describe people as tall, average-sized, and short. However, in developing comfortable chairs, for example, more refined measures, such as the inches scale, are needed.

Such a continuous dimensional approach, although entirely understandable, tends to prevent the detection of qualitative discontinuities. The fact that one can measure the size of all people with a foot rule does not imply the nonexistence of qualitative distinctions in height like those resulting from such conditions as pituitary gigantism or cretinism.

We wish to outline a program for the development of a diagnostic system appropriate to our present stage of psychiatric knowledge.

THEORY OF DIAGNOSIS

Most psychiatrists utilize the diagnostic system without attempting to think through the logical and scientific issues implied in the use of this device. Anyone attending the usual diagnostic staff conference cannot but be confounded by the general incoherence of the proceedings.

An exact scientific description of a complex system requires the ability to dissect a phenomenon into its components and then to synthesize the phenomenon through knowledge of the components, of their interrelationships, and of the laws governing them. Except for rather simple physical systems, such an ideal is not attained in a very broad range of scientific study. Dynamic diagnostic formulations attempt to explain the manifest psychiatric illness as the superficial aspect of the interacting underlying variables. Unfortunately, the evidence for such formulations is often compatible with several opposing views, and there is no method available for determining which, if any, is correct.

Studies of humans suffer from a lack of precise knowledge of components, relationships, or laws. Therefore much scientific study of humans consists of variations on "black box" procedures. That is, the attempt to dissect the phenomenon into its significant parts is deferred. Instead, one attempts to discover systematic relationships among various inputs and various organismal effects—eg, digitalis, and slowing of the pulse rate; diuretics, and relief of edema. Analysis of the observed regularities may then lead to hypotheses concerning the significant components (heart, kidneys, etc.) of the black box and the applicable laws.

At a still more primitive stage of scientific analysis, one is interested in detecting regularities in outputs for which there is no knowledge of the relevant input. This method allows the labeling of regularly occurring, complex states, thereby increasing communication and providing a focus for further work. For instance, one might notice that among a group of people there is a sudden outbreak of rice-water diarrhea, vomiting, muscular cramps, dehydration, anuria, and collapse. These symptoms may be grouped into a syndrome and labeled "cholera," without knowledge of causation or input.

A debate might easily start: Is cholera a distinct disease with a unitary etiology, or is it simply a variant of the acute diarrheas whose particular clinical features are due to some pathoplastic variation in the constitution of those affected? For instance, do patients with rice-water stools have a different illness from that of patients with dysentery marked by stools with blood, pus, and mucus? One might even take the stand that defecation is part of life. Since diarrhea is simply excessive defecation, it should not be considered a disease at all but rather a style of life.

Several possibilities exist for resolving this issue: One might attempt to show that there were markedly different phenomenal patterns within the diarrheas. For instance, rice-water diarrhea is regularly associated with a marked leukocytosis, whereas bloody diarrhea is often associated with a leukopenia or low-grade leukocytosis. However, intermediate cases do exist, and one might argue that these are simply two extremes of a continuum rather than qualitatively discrete syndromes.

Or, one might attempt to relate the symptom pattern to course and outcome, showing that cholera is 50% fatal in adults whereas dysenteries are hardly ever fatal in adults.

One might defer to the differential effects of empiric treatments. For instance, sulfonamides are regularly effective with the dysenteries but only slightly, if at all, effective with cholera. This clinical difference would seem to be powerful evidence of a true biologic difference between the two syndromes. But, even here, an occasional case of cholera may seem to respond to sulfonamides, whereas an occasional case of dysentery may not respond.

It seems plain, then, that a distinction between the syndromes can be supported with varying degrees of confidence by studies of symptom pattern, prognosis, and response to treatment. Nonetheless, it is always possible to take the stand that these patterns are simply variations on a common theme and should not be dignified as separate diseases.

Two other possibilities exist for determining whether these syndromes are actually discrete. One may analyze the pathophysiologic process that underlies the symptoms. For instance, on sigmoidoscope examination, patients with cholera show surprisingly normal viscera, whereas those with dysentery show an acute inflammatory process marked by hyperemia and ulceration. This difference in pathophysiologic process argues strongly for a difference in causation and therefore a qualitative distinction between the syndromes.

However, the most convincing distinction in syndromal analysis is made by etiology. If it can be determined that the cholera syndrome is necessarily induced by infection with the *vibrio comma,* whereas dysentery is caused by the *shigella* group of organisms, we can then state firmly that we have two separate diseases, characterized by distinct etiologies, pathophysiologies, pathoplastic factors, treatment responses, and prognoses. This is the ideal diagnosis of clinical medicine.

It is evident from this discussion that analysis of psychiatric phenomena is, in principle, similar to the general problems that medicine has confronted throughout its history. In psychiatry we rarely know etiology and practically never know pathophysiology. Therefore we are at the level of forming descriptive categorizations, which hopefully allow for valid predictions. This approach does not prejudge the questions of single versus multiple etiologic factors, or discount the adaptive role of the organism in shaping the syndrome.

One must distinguish the defining characteristics of a class (the reliability question) from the correlates of class membership (the validity question).

A classificatory system is *reliable* insofar as the defining characteristics of a class are measurable and communicable so that different observers will classify subjects (diagnose illnesses) similarly. In an attempt to specify unequivocal classifications on the basis of multiple descriptive measures, several computer-based logical decision-tree procedures have been developed.[6-8] Spitzer and Endicott[6] and Nathan[7] utilize an *a priori* diagnostic approach. Klein, Honigfeld, and Feldman[8] developed an inductive procedure that arrives at a decision tree from diagnostic behavior.

A classificatory system is *valid* insofar as it allows correct statements that extend beyond the defining characteristics of the class, about the members of the class. For instance, one might establish a diagnostic class "Retarded Depression," on the basis of certain defining characteristics derived from patients' histories, affective complaints, and psychomotor behaviors. However, if one could then predict correctly that such patients would respond better to electroconvulsive therapy than other patients, one would be demonstrating that this diagnostic system had validity. In this case, the criterion of class validity is prediction of treatment response. One might also have predicted that such patients eventually would spontaneously recover without any specific therapeutic intervention. The correctness of this prediction would demonstrate diagnostic validity in terms of prognosis and illness course. One might further claim that there is a high incidence of affective disorders in the parents of such patients. The correctness of this prediction would support the validity of this classification in terms of familial phenomena. A diagnostic classification that validly predicts familial characteristics, course, prognosis, and treatment response would seem likely to be a specific discrete syndrome that reflects some common etiologic factor or set of factors.

Making Syndromes Useful

Therefore, instead of etiologic diagnoses of illness, various syndromal groupings of historic features, illness course, and examinational traits must be provisionally used, with the understanding that similar syndromes may have diverse etiologies. Even the most widely used psychiatric nosology in the United States, the *Diagnostic and Statistical Manual, Mental Disorders* of the American Psychiatric Association,[9, 10] does not take a consistent stand on this issue. The diagnostic categories are at times purely descriptive (eg, compulsive personality), mixed descriptive and presumed etiologic (eg, emotionally unstable personality), or predominantly etiologic (eg, psychophysiologic disorder). If the dynamic and etiologic sequences stipulated in this manual are considered unproved, one is frequently at a loss when attempting to use its classification.

The 1968 revision of this manual (DSM II) is as yet untested. However, it appears to be a distinct improvement, since there is a marked decrease in etiologic inference as a component of syndrome definition.[10] Nonetheless, this renewed emphasis on objective description has been attacked as a reversion to a simplistic disease theory.

Because of the lack of etiologic information, all syndrome categorizations are provisional and open to radical revision. Nonetheless, certain improvements are possible over the present slipshod state. One dubious method that has achieved considerable interest consists of the systematic recording of a wide variety of traits in psychiatric patients, producing individual profiles. These profiles are then computer-inspected to see whether similar profiles may be clustered, reflecting naturally occurring types.

This seems quite reasonable, and approximates clinical practice wherein certain salient combinations, such as retardation and depression, delusions and hallucinations, phobic-anxious states and depersonalization, have been noted. Unfortunately, this apparently objective syndromal approach demands the ability to define the similarity of patterns. Although many mathematical attempts have been made to produce such an all-purpose similarity measure, there is no unanimity among the experts, and we believe that there is a basic arbitrariness to this method that renders it forever unlikely to do more than demonstrate the obvious. In particular, good clustering requires a foreknowledge of the traits that distinguish the clusters. Irrelevant traits prevent the detection of clusters.

An alternative method exists that appears more useful. Rather than search for natural trait clusters that fall into nearly discrete syndromes, it is possible to determine those combinations of psychiatric traits that allow for maximally effective prediction of some criterion variable, such as prognosis or response to medication. Essentially this was the method of Kraepelin. He isolated, from the welter of clinical traits, those that were regularly associated with a deteriorative course, and thus defined dementia praecox. The strength of this method is that the syndromes are open to test; they either predict and have at least pragmatic justification, or they don't and have at best esthetic value. Much current activity actually represents a reversion from the premature Bleulerian emphasis on discerning the inferred processes underlying groups of symptoms to the Kraepelinian model of attempting to delineate those trait complexes that allow maximum predictive ability.

Therefore, in the absence of etiologic knowledge, the best approach is to segregate statistically the natural groupings of developmental, historic, symptomatic, and examinational findings that convey prognostic or treatment relevant information. Dynamic formulations that have demonstrable prognostic or treatment relevant implications fall quite naturally into this model. Hopefully, these functionally valuable syndromes may also be relatively homogeneous for etiology, and therefore of value in etiologic research.

REVIEW OF RESEARCH AT HILLSIDE HOSPITAL RELEVANT TO DIAGNOSIS

At Hillside Hospital (Glen Oaks, New York), we found that diagnosis was essential in our studies of prognosis and response to psychopharmacologic agents. Also, comparative studies of diagnostic and appropriate comparison groups have given us some leads concerning the possible genesis of these conditions.

PSYCHOPHARMACOLOGY

Our pilot studies with imipramine (Tofrānil) and the phenothiazines indicated that the distinction between schizophrenia and the affective disorders was of key importance in predicting drug effect.[11] These pilot studies were followed by a double-blind, fixed-dosage, random-assignment, placebo-controlled study of chlorpromazine (Thorazine) and imipramine in a heterogeneous group of more than 300 non-chronic voluntary psychiatric inpatients. Analysis of behavioral ratings indicated that depressive and schizophrenic subgroups demonstrated different rating scale patterns of drug effect.[12]

We further showed that patients diagnostically characterized by the sudden onset of episodic anxiety, with fear of unaccompanied travel and phobic dependent manipulations, showed a diagnosis specific response to antidepressant medication; their panic attacks were alleviated. However, a period of desensitization was required to alleviate their anticipatory anxiety. Phenothiazines exacerbated their condition. A double-blind clinical study indicated that these were not placebo effects.

Two clinical subcategories were demonstrated. The first group had had a chronically high level of separation anxiety since childhood, and developed panic attacks under conditions of separation or bereavement. The second group had unremarkable developmental histories, and developed attacks in a context of altered endocrine functions.[13] These studies demonstrated a clear-cut relationship between diagnosis and drug effect.

Further investigating the utility of diagnosis in predicting drug effects, we were able to demonstrate that other specific drug-diagnosis interactions and the prediction of global outcome by diagnosis were possible.[14] The factors predictive of drug effects broadened our conception of diagnosis to include developmental history and activation status.

To refine further the relationship of drug effect to diagnosis, we devised an alternative measuring device to Global Improvement Scales. Here patients were assigned to Qualitative Outcome Categories on the basis of the configuration of multiple changes. We demonstrated that this outcome typology was equal or superior to the Global Improvement Scale in detecting the differences between drugs and placebo. Moreover, by using the author's diagnostic schema as well as the qualitative outcome typology, the prediction of specific drug-induced qualitative outcomes by diagnosis was demonstrated.[15] This was impossible using an all-purpose conglomerate Global Improvement Scale.

Because of the difficulties in reliably assigning patients to either diagnoses or qualitative outcome classes, a series of explorations was conducted concerning the possibility of computerizing this process.[8, 16-18] The decision-tree method that was developed uses behavioral scales derived from interview, ward behavior, self-ratings, etc., as basic data, as well as an overall diagnostic judgment made by senior diagnosticians. The problem is how to use the scales so that the diagnosis can be reliably approximated in a fashion that makes clinical sense.

We have developed a computer program that inductively generates a decision tree utilizing the behavioral data, terminating in a diagnostic classification. One possible merit of this procedure is that it does not depend upon an *a priori* system of logical decisions, but imitates the actual behavior of a diagnostician. Preliminary studies[8] have shown that decision-tree diagnoses parallel clinical diagnoses in their ability to predict drug effects. However, considerable further refinement is still necessary.

A review of the scientific psychopharmacologic treatment literature found that the major drawback to generalizing from individual studies is the lack of specification of the patient sample.[1] This widely recognized fact has led to a tremendous resurgence of interest in the possibility of methodical psychiatric description and diagnosis. Our recent book (*Diagnosis and Drug Treatment of Psychiatric Disorders*) attempts to integrate what is presently known about diagnosis and psychopharmacologic treatment.[1]

A review of Hillside Hospital studies on diagnosis and reaction to drug treatment led to the following formulations:

1. Certain psychiatric illnesses (manic-depressive and hyperactive paranoid) are primarily caused by deranged affective-activation mechanisms and have minimal secondary, functionally autonomous, symptomatic reverberations. These illnesses have naturally occurring, complete remissions, and also respond best to psychotropic drugs.

2. Other psychiatric illnesses (periodic-anxious states, agitated depressions in obsessional states, emotionally unstable character disorders, and the schizophrenias) are characterized both by affective-activation disorders and a secondary residue that persists after the termination of the affective derangement. Psychotropic drugs

again mimic the natural course of the illness, since these illnesses are characterized by naturally occurring remissions with persistent secondary symptoms.

3. Other psychiatric illnesses that are not characterized by a primary activation-affective disorder are refractory to psychotropic agents. However, histrionic-hysterical states and chronic anticipatory anxiety states require special differentiation, since their affective difficulties appear to have a different origin.

4. Psychotropic drugs may work by normalizing deranged affective-activation mechanisms. To the degree that a psychiatric illness is due to such deranged activation mechanisms, the drug effects will mimic the processes of natural remission.[19]

Diagnosis and Prognosis

The ability to make a firm prognosis on the basis of diagnosis is one of the clearest assurances of diagnostic validity. It was on this basis that Kraepelin erected the distinction between dementia praecox and manic-depressive disease. This distinction has been blurred by the Bleulerian emphasis on diagnosing schizophrenia via the recognition of certain basic psychopathologic defects. Bleuler was not concerned with developing diagnostic categories with prognostic significance. Therefore it should be no surprise that his category of schizophrenia has less prognostic worth than Kraepelin's category of dementia praecox. In recent years the value of diagnosis for prognostic studies has been specifically attacked. Several theoreticians, notably Zigler and Phillips,[4] have proposed prognostic indices whose utility cuts across diagnostic boundaries and renders diagnosis irrelevant to prognosis.

However, in our follow-up studies, we noted that diagnosis was definitely of prognostic import.[20-22] Further, these studies indicated the importance of early socialization patterns, affective instability, and age at onset of illness as diagnostically related prognosticators.[5, 23, 24]

We studied the relationship of the Zigler and Phillips Social Competence Scale to outcome, to test whether it is a prognostic index that cuts across diagnosis. We found that among schizophrenic patients, social competence was positively related to two of five indices of posthospital outcome: incidence and frequency of rehospitalization. However, among nonschizophrenic patients the re-

lationship between incidence of rehospitalization and social competence was not statistically significant. With regard to frequency of
rehospitalization a surprising, significant negative relationship was
obtained.[25]

Further analysis showed that the prognostic value of the Zigler
and Phillips scale for schizophrenia was based entirely on its relationship to age at first psychiatric treatment contact.[5] This indicated the significance that both age at first-treatment contact and
social competence were functions of diagnosis rather than panpsychopathologic indices.

It is certainly possible that certain indices, such as intelligence,
may be of prognostic value both within and across diagnostic
categories. It is our contention, however, that diagnosis has been
prematurely discarded as a potent prognostic variable that deter-
mines the functional meaning of social and demographic variables.

Distinguishing Features of Diagnostic Groups

An enormous number of studies have demonstrated a host of physiologic, biochemical, psychologic, demographic, developmental, and
other differences between different psychiatric diagnostic groups
and normals. The problem with most such studies is that the
diagnostic differences are confounded by differences in age, sex,
education, social class, treatment history, hospitalization experience,
diet, exposure to toxins, and other such factors. To demonstrate such
differences validly requires the most meticulous attention to match-
ing patients and comparison groups.

We have shown differences between diagnostic subgroups with
relationship to Rorschach responses,[26] EEG,[27] mecholyl response,[28]
RAI uptake,[29] and "soft" behavioral organic signs.[30] However,
the objections to the diagnostic comparisons itemized above hold for
these studies also. For instance, we showed that the mecholyl
responses of 338 psychiatric patients were correlated with psychiatric diagnosis, age, and base blood pressure. However, when age
was partialed out, the correlation between diagnosis and mecholyl
response was no longer significant.[28]

To deal with the problem of control, we have recently become
interested in the possibility of using the patient's siblings as comparison groups. Obviously, the siblings are as well matched as one
can expect with regard to family background, education, social

class, and general life experience. Such studies also afford an opportunity for measuring familial concordance.[31-33]

CONCLUSION

We hope we have demonstrated that systematic patient description and classification is crucial to the development of a rational approach to treatment and prognosis. Further, classifications that validly predict treatment response and prognosis should foster the development of etiologic studies. The recent development of measurement and computer techniques affords us a tremendous opportunity to develop such methods systematically.

"Generally, it can be said that the use of statistics is an admission of defeat by the scientist. It means that we understand so little about the underlying mechanism that we are forced to use chance mechanisms and averaging techniques."[34] This is exactly our present position. Our goal is to progress from statistical prediction to a structural-functional-etiologic body of knowledge that allows precise analysis of the individual case. The unwarranted wishful-thinking presumption that we have already attained this level of understanding of psychiatric illnesses has paralyzed the appropriate development of data-gathering and treatment-measuring programs.

Advancing psychiatric knowledge requires developing large multidisciplinary teams to dovetail the behavioral and symptomatic effects of treatment with the longitudinal intricacies of patients' history, thinking, and affective regulation. However, the need for such teams has not received wide consideration because it is incongruous with the prevailing organization of psychiatric and psychopharmacologic research. Most psychopharmacologic research involves short-term programs where patients are initially examined, then treated, and examined again, by a variety of raters. Prolonged clinical contact with study patients by research clinicians occurs rarely, despite the fact that the experienced clinician, given the opportunity to utilize his skills, is our most sensitive cluster analytic device. Present programs militate against any such opportunity, as do multihospital studies, which should be considered the product of administrative necessity rather than scientific value.

It should be plain that both the technical flaws in present studies and the possible goals of future studies can best be answered by the development of large, comprehensive psychiatric research facilities.

This is not a new idea, since a number of small clinical research centers have developed, funded by the National Institute of Mental Health and largely confined to 20-bed units. This small-scale operation enforces small-scale work. Although brilliant pilot work, especially in the metabolic-biochemical area, can be done with only a few patients, the diagnostic and treatment assessment goals outlined above need larger populations, approximating 200 patients.

The purpose of such a research facility would be to determine which patients respond best to which therapies or combination of therapies. This can be definitively answered only by a series of studies that revolve around controlled random assignment to treatment and long-term follow-up via a continued-care program.[35, 36] Staffing such centers presents another problem. Existing centers usually are run by one to three senior people and a moderate-sized group of junior professionals in transit to senior positions elsewhere. The complex studies outlined above require the development of a large, integrated senior staff sharing a primary interest in better patient classification and treatment evaluation. Such a facility should offer tenure to its senior staff, as well as the financial remuneration that would make these positions competitive with the rewards of private practice. University affiliation would be desirable both for an increase in status and for the recruitment of new personnel. However, for such a facility to be successful in its programmatic mission, it would have to maintain considerable autonomy in order to avoid being diverted to the pet projects of department chairmen.

The emphasis on treatment evaluation would require the easy availability of the entire gamut of accepted therapies, plus a high level of clinical practice.

No doubt, this would be an expensive undertaking. We estimate that in 1969 a 200-bed research inpatient facility, with a well-developed continued-care program for all patients and an active outpatient clinic, would require an annual minimum of five million dollars. If the average length of stay was six months, 1,200 patients could be studied in three years. It is clear, however, that without such a facility we can arrive at only piecemeal answers to the many complicated questions of psychiatric care. The total spent on limited treatment-evaluation studies far exceeds the cost of running several facilities of this nature.

Such facilities can lay the foundations for the eventual development of individualized structural-functional-etiologic diagnoses, with clear-cut prognostic and treatment implications.

REFERENCES

1. Klein, D. F., and Davis, J. M.: *Diagnosis and Drug Treatment of Psychiatric Disorders,* Baltimore, Md.: Williams and Wilkins, 1969.
2. Menninger, K.: *The Vital Balance,* New York: Viking Press, 1963.
3. Szasz, T.: *Myth of Mental Illness,* New York: Harper & Bros., 1961.
4. Zigler, E., and Phillips, L.: Social Competence and Outcome in Psychiatric Disorder, *J. Abn. Soc. Psychol.,* 63:264–271, 1961.
5. Rosen, B., Klein, D. F., Levenstein, S., and Shahinian, S. P.: Social Competence and Posthospital Outcome, *Arch. Gen. Psychiat.,* 19:165–170, 1968.
6. Spitzer, R. L., and Endicott, J. Diagno, II: Further Developments in a Computer Program for Psychiatric Diagnosis, *Amer. J. Psychiat.,* 125 (supp.):7, 12, 1969.
7. Nathan, P. E.: *Cues, Decisions and Diagnoses,* New York: Academic Press, 1967.
8. Klein, D. F., Honigfeld, G., and Feldman, S.: Prediction of Drug Effects by Diagnostic Decision Tree, *Dis. Nerv. Syst.,* 29 (suppl.): 159–187, 1968.
9. *Diagnostic and Statistical Manual, Mental Disorders,* Washington, D.C.: American Psychiatric Association, 1952.
10. *Diagnostic and Statistical Manual, Mental Disorders,* ed. 2, Washington, D.C.: American Psychiatric Association, 1968.
11. Klein, D. F., and Fink, M.: Psychiatric Reaction Patterns to Imipramine, *Amer. J. Psychiat.,* 119:432–438, 1962.
12. Klein, D. F., and Fink, M.: Multiple Item Factors as Change Measures in Psychopharmacology, *Psychopharmacologia,* 4:43–52, 1963.
13. Klein, D. F.: Delineation of Two Drug-Responsive Anxiety Syndromes, *Psychopharmacologia,* 5:397–408, 1964.
14. Klein, D. F.: Importance of Psychiatric Diagnosis in Prediction of Clinical Drug Effects, *Arch. Gen. Psychiat.,* 16:118–126, 1967.
15. Klein, D. F.: Psychiatric Diagnosis and Typology of Clinical Drug Effects, *Psychopharmacologia,* 13:359–386, 1968.
16. Feldman, S., Klein, D. F., and Honigfeld, G.: Analysis of Drug Therapy Response in Psychiatric Patients Using a Sequential Screening Decision Tree Technique, *Biometrics.* In press.
17. Honigfeld, G. H., Klein, D. F., and Feldman, S.: Prediction of Psychopharmacologic Effect in Man: Development and Validation of a Computerized Diagnostic Decision Tree, *Comput. Biomed. Res.* In press.
18. Klein, D. F., Honigfeld, G., and Feldman, S.: "Prediction of Drug Effect by Successive Screening Decision Tree Diagnostic Technique," in May, P. R. A., in Wittenborn, J. R. (eds.): *Psychotropic Drug Response: Advances in Prediction,* Springfield, Ill.: Charles C. Thomas. In press.
19. Klein, D. F.: "Diagnosis and Pattern of Reaction to Drug Treatment: Clinically Derived Formulations," in Katz, N. M., Cole, J. O., and Barton, W. E. (eds.): *Role of Methodology of Classification in Psychiatry and Psychopathology,* Washington, D.C.: U.S. Government Printing Office, 466–483, 1968.

244 New Approaches to Research and Education

20. Levenstein, S., Klein, D. F., and Pollack, M.: Follow-up Study of Formerly Hospitalized Voluntary Psychiatric Patients: First Two Years, *Amer. J. Psychiat.*, 122:1102–1109, 1966.
21. Pollack, M., Levenstein, S., and Klein, D. F.: Three Year Posthospital Follow-up of Psychiatric Patients: First Hospitalization in Adolescence vs. Adulthood, *Internat. J. Child Psychiat.*, 33:224–225, 1966.
22. Quitkin, F. M., and Klein, D. F.: Follow-up of Treatment Failure: Psychosis and Character Disorders, *Amer. J. Psychiat.*, 124:499–505, 1967.
23. Pollack, M., Levenstein, S., and Klein, D. F.: Three Year Posthospital Follow-up of Adolescent and Adult Schizophrenics, *Amer. J. Orthopsychiat.*, 38:94–109, 1968.
24. Gittelman-Klein, R. K., and Klein, D. F.: Relationship Between Premorbid Asocial Adjustment and Prognosis in Schizophrenia, *J. Psychiat. Res.* In press.
25. Rosen, B., Klein, D. F., Levenstein, S., and Shahinian, S.: Social Competence and Posthospital Outcome Among Schizophrenic and Non-Schizophrenic Psychiatric Patients, *J. Abnorm. Psychol.* In press.
26. Belmont, I., Birch, H. G., Klein, D. F., and Pollack, M.: Perceptual Evidence of CNS Dysfunction in Schizophrenia, *Arch. Gen. Psychiat.*, 10:395–408, 1964.
27. Kennard, M. A., Pollack, M., and Klein, D. F.: EEG Qualities in Group of Young Adult Hospitalized Psychiatric Patients, *Rec. Adv. Biol. Psychiat.*, 8:277–282, 1966.
28. Blumberg, A. G., and Klein, D. F.: Age, Base Blood Pressure, Diagnosis, and Mecholyl Test Response, *Psychosom. Med.*, 28:789–794, 1966.
29. Blumberg, A. G., and Klein, D. F.: Psychiatric Diagnosis, Activation and Radioactive Iodine Uptake, *Arch. Gen. Psychiat.*, 18:601–611, 1968.
30. Quitkin, F. M., and Klein, D. F.: Two Behavioral Syndromes in Young Adults Related to Possible Minimal Brain Dysfunction, *J. Psychiat. Res.* In press.
31. Pollack, M., Woerner, M. G., Goldberg, P., and Klein, D. F.: Psychopathology and Gender Concordance in the Siblings of Schizophrenic and Nonschizophrenic Psychiatric Patients, *Arch. Gen. Psychiat.* In press.
32. Pollack, M., Woerner, M. G., and Klein, D. F.: "Comparison of Childhood Characteristics of Schizophrenics, Personality Disorders and Their Siblings," in Roff, M., and Ricks, D. (eds.): *Life History Factors and Psychopathology*, Minneapolis: University of Minnesota Press. In press.
33. Woerner, M. G., Pollack, M., and Klein, D. F.: Birth Weight and Length in Schizophrenics, Personality Disorders and Their Siblings. Uupublished manuscript.
34. Bellman, R.: *Some Vistas of Modern Mathematics*, Lexington, Ky.: University of Kentucky Press, 1968.
35. Gittelman, R. K., Klein, D. F., and Pollack, M.: Effects of Psychotropic Drugs on Long-Term Adjustment: A Review, *Psychopharmacologia*, 5:317–338, 1964.
36. Gittelman-Klein, R. K., and Klein, D. F.: Long-Term Effects of Antipsychotic Agents: A Review, from Proceedings of American College of Neuropsychopharmacology, Puerto Rico, 1967.

13

Social Competence
and Posthospital Outcome*

by BERNARD ROSEN,

DONALD F. KLEIN,

SIDNEY LEVENSTEIN,

and SIROON P. SHAHINIAN

Hillside Hospital studies of prognosis have emphasized the utility of psychiatric diagnosis[1] and age at onset of illness.[2] Zigler and Phillips,[3] utilizing a different approach, suggest the central role of personal and social maturity. In their view, as an individual ages, he passes through successive levels of maturity. At each level, society presents a complex of tasks with which the individual is expected to cope. The higher the maturational level attained, the greater the resources the individual should have to enable him to cope successfully with society's expectations.

Since for every maturational level there exist normal adaptive patterns, as well as pathologic deviations from these patterns, in the opinion of Zigler and Phillips psychopathology can be viewed as representing various inappropriate methods of coping with specific tasks appropriate to the age or expected level of maturation.

* This study was supported in part by PHS research grants MH-10191 and MH-08004 from the NIMH and by a grant provided by the Board of Directors, Hillside Hospital. Mr. Robert E. Patton, Director of the Biostatistics Division of the New York State Department of Mental Hygiene, made records available.

Published in the *Archives of General Psychiatry*, Vol. 19, August 1969, pp. 165–170, and reproduced with permission.

The higher the maturity level attained prior to the onset of illness, the greater the resources for undoing inappropriate (pathologic) solutions for social tasks, and the better the prognosis.

To test the validity of this approach, the concept of Premorbid Social Competence (defined by a scale consisting of age, intelligence, education, occupation, employment history, and marital status) was employed by Zigler and Phillips as an "approximation of personal and social maturity."[3] Although Phillips[4] defines the Social Competence Scale as reflecting "socio-economic potential and the likelihood that age and sex role expectations will be fulfilled," supporting data are not presented. An examination of the scoring instructions[3, 5] raises questions concerning the construct validity of this scale. The term "Premorbid" is defined[6] as "occurring before the development of disease." Zigler and Phillips did not place this restriction upon the variables used as criteria for measuring social competence. The inclusion of behavior occurring at the point of, as well as immediately preceding, hospitalization suggests that the Zigler and Phillips' scale may be confounded with measures of morbid social competence. Furthermore, an examination of the variables in the scale leads one to question if it is applicable even as a measure of morbid social competence. Although education, occupation, employment history, and marital status may be considered appropriate measures of social attainment among adults, their relevance is questionable for patients who have just begun their adult careers. For adolescent patients, these variables are clearly inappropriate. A 17-year-old high school student would be rated "low" in social competence, according to Zigler and Phillips' criteria, regardless of intelligence, school performance, or ability to socialize and form meaningful relationships.

The inclusion of the variable age as a specific item, coupled with additional items where the possibility of a "high" score (reflective of "high" social competence) is limited to adults, suggests that the social competence scale is, with regard to its relationship to prognosis, reducible to age. When one considers that Zigler and Phillips limited their 1961 sample to patients who had never been previously hospitalized,[3] then the age variable is in fact age of first psychiatric hospitalization, which may be closely related to age at onset of illness.

This paper questions the interpretation offered by Zigler and Phillips[3] that the relationship found between their scale and post-hospital outcome demonstrates the existence of a relationship between premorbid social competence and prognosis. It is our contention that their findings can be entirely accounted for by the relationship between their social competence scale and age at onset of illness.

METHOD

The sample studied consisted of 166 psychiatric patients described previously.[1,7] The patients were studied intensively while they were inpatients at Hillside Hospital; they were discharged between June 1961 and May 1962. Of the original sample of 176 patients, 10 could not be followed up and were excluded from this study. Mean age at the time of hospitalization was 32.5 years; the female: male ratio was 2:1. The majority of patients were high school graduates and had completed at least one year of post-high school education. One third of the sample had been previously hospitalized in a psychiatric institution. Hospitalization at Hillside Hospital averaged eight months. Socio-economic status was measured by Hollingshead's Two Factor Index of Social Position. Socio-economic classes I through V characterized respectively 9%, 17%, 29%, 36%, and 9% of the sample.

Patients were diagnosed by the research psychiatrist according to criteria presented previously.[8] The sample was diagnostically heterogeneous; 81 patients were diagnosed as schizophrenic. The remainder (N = 85) consisted primarily of patients with affective and character disorders.

Follow-up interviews were conducted after the second and third year following discharge from Hillside Hospital. Each patient, as well as a close relative with an intimate knowledge of the patient during the period surveyed, was interviewed separately by a specially trained psychiatric social worker. All patients who had moved from the New York City area were interviewed by experienced local psychiatric social workers in the patient's new location. Additional data were received from treatment sources utilized by the patients during the follow-up period. Psychiatric rehospitalizations were further checked through the Biostatistics Division of the New York State Department of Mental Hygiene.

The social competence measure employed was identical to that specified by Zigler and Phillips[3]; it consists of the variables age, intelligence (Wechsler Adult Intelligence Scale "WAIS"), occupation, employment history, marital status, and education. The variables were categorized, and total social competence scores were computed by the methods described by Zigler and Phillips.[3] To form high and low social competence groups, the distribution of social competence scores was divided as close to the median as was possible. Patients with a mean social competence score of 1.17 or more were considered high. The remaining patients comprised the low competence group.

Because of the problems involved in reliably determining the exact age at onset of illness, age at first psychiatric treatment contact was used as an estimate. The distribution of this variable was also divided as close to the median as possible. The outcome measure employed was the Incidence of Psychiatric Rehospitalization occurring during the three-year follow-up period (two patients who had never been rehospitalized but who had committed suicide were included in the rehospitalized group).

RESULTS

The cross-validation of the Social Competence Scale on our sample indicated that a significantly higher proportion of low competence patients (54 patients or 62.1%) were rehospitalized, as compared to 26% or 32.9% of the patients in the high competence group ($\chi^2 = 14.10$, P<0.001).

The results obtained with age at first psychiatric treatment contact were similar to those obtained using the Social Competence Scale. A significantly higher proportion of patients who first entered psychiatric treatment prior to the age of 23 (55% or 64.6%) were rehospitalized, as compared to 25% or 30.9% of those who were older at the time of their first psychiatric treatment contact ($\chi^2 = 19.02$, P<0.001). In addition, the Social Competence Scale and age at first psychiatric treatment contact were significantly related to each other ($\phi = 0.71$, P<0.001).

To determine the joint effect of social competence and age at first psychiatric treatment contact on the incidence of rehospitalization, a two-way analysis of variance of proportions (using an arc sine data transformation) was performed according to the methods for unequal subclasses.[9, 10] From the data in Table 1, it is evident that the predictive power of Zigler and Phillips' Social Competence Scale is due to its relationship with age at first psychiatric treatment contact. A significantly higher proportion of the patients treated prior to the age of 23 were rehospitalized, regardless of level of

TABLE 1

Social Competence and Age at First Psychiatric Treatment*

| | Age of First Psychiatric Treatment | | | |
| | 0–22 | | 23+ | |
Social Competence	Hospitalized (Percent)	Total (No.)	Hospitalized (Percent)	Total (No.)
Low	64.9	74	46.2	13
High	63.6	11	27.9	68

| | Summary of Analysis of Variance | | | | |
Source	Sum of Squares	df	Mean Square	F-Ratio	P
Age	4968.90	1	4968.90	6.05	< 0.025
Competence	781.97	1	781.97	0.95	NS
Interaction	520.38	1	520.38	0.63	NS
Error	–	∞	820.70	–	–

* Incidence of rehospitalization.

social competence, than patients in the older group ($P<0.025$). The insignificant interaction effect indicates that the differences in rehospitalization rates between low (46.2%) and high (27.9%) social competence patients within the older group are within the limits of chance variation.

Recognizing that the above results may be confounded by the fact that age at first psychiatric treatment contact is highly correlated ($\phi = 0.81$, $P<0.001$) with the age variable that is part of Zigler and Phillips' Social Competence Scale, a further analysis of the data was performed excluding the age variable from the Social Competence Scale. Social competence scores were recomputed using the five remaining variables—marital status, intelligence, education, occupation, and employment history. The sample was again divided as close to the median of this new distribution as possible. Patients with a mean social competence score of 1.20 or more were considered "high" in social competence. The remaining patients comprised the "low" competence group.

The modified Social Competence Scale was also effective in predicting incidence of rehospitalization. Again, a significantly higher proportion of low competence patients were rehospitalized (48% or

62.3%) as compared to 32% or 36% of the patients in the "high" competence group who were also rehospitalized ($\chi^2 = 11.51$, $P<0.001$). However, even with the age variable excluded, the modified Social Competence Scale was still significantly related to age at first psychiatric treatment contact ($\phi = 0.47$, $P < 0.001$).

The results of the second analysis of variance were consistent with those presented previously. Again a significantly higher proportion of the patients treated prior to the age of 23 were rehospital-

TABLE 2

Social Competence Less Age and Age at First Psychiatric Treatment*

Social competence less age	Age of First Psychiatric Treatment			
	0–22		23+	
	Hospitalized (Percent)	Total (No.)	Hospitalized (Percent)	Total (No.)
Low	69.5	59	38.9	18
High	53.8	26	38.6	63

Summary of Analysis of Variance					
Source	Sum of Squares	df	Mean Square	F-Ratio	P
Age	8434.10	1	8434.10	10.28	<0.005
Competence	2045.76	1	2045.76	2.49	NS
Interaction	71.04	1	71.04	0.08	NS
Error	–	∞	820.70	–	–

* Incidence of rehospitalization.

ized, regardless of level of social competence, than of patients in the "older" group ($P<0.005$). Again, there was no significant interaction effect.

The results presented thus far are for a diagnostically heterogeneous group of patients. Although Zigler and Phillips contend that an identical relationship between social competence and prognosis is found in both a schizophrenic and nonschizophrenic hospital population,[3,5] supporting evidence is not presented. In a previous paper[11] we demonstrated that although the Zigler and Phillips' Social Competence Scale was related to posthospital outcome among schizophrenic patients, this relationship was not found among nonschizophrenic patients. To clarify the relationship between the present findings and diagnosis, we analyzed the data in Table 2 separately for schizophrenic and nonschizophrenic patients.

With regard to schizophrenic patients, a significantly positive relationship was found between the incidence of rehospitalization and the modified Social Competence Scale ($\chi^2 = 9.61$, P<0.01) as

TABLE 3

Schizophrenic Patients, Social Competence Less Age and Age at First Psychiatric Treatment*

	Age at First Psychiatric Treatment			
	0–22		23+	
Social competence less age	Hospitalized (Percent)	Total (No.)	Hospitalized (Percent)	Total (No.)
Low	80.0	40	40.0	5
High	69.2	13	26.1	23

Summary of Analysis of Variance					
Source	Sum of Squares	df	Mean Square	F-Ratio	P
Age	8030.06	1	8030.06	9.78	<0.005
Competence	793.84	1	793.84	0.97	NS
Interaction	5.32	1	5.32	0.01	NS
Error	–	∞	820.70	–	–

* Incidence of rehospitalization.

well as age at first psychiatric treatment contact ($\chi^2 = 18.25$, P<0.001). The results of the analysis of variance (Table 3) were again consistent with those presented above. Again a significantly higher proportion of the patients treated prior to the age of 23 were rehospitalized regardless of level of social competence (P<0.005).

For nonschizophrenic patients the relationship between incidence of rehospitalization and either the modified Social Competence Scale or age at first psychiatric treatment contact was not significant.

COMMENTS

The results of the present study confirm the findings of Zigler and Phillips[3] that a positive relationship exists between their Social

TABLE 4

Nonschizophrenic Patients, Social Competence Less Age and Age at First Psychiatric Treatment*

| Social competence less age | Age at First Psychiatric Treatment | | | |
| | 0–22 | | 23+ | |
	Hospitalized (Percent)	Total (No.)	Hospitalized (Percent)	Total (No.)
Low	47.4	19	38.5	13
High	38.5	13	30.0	40

| Summary of Analysis of Variance | | | | | |
Source	Sum of Squares	df	Mean Square	F-Ratio	P
Age	464.64	1	464.64	0.57	NS
Competence	464.64	1	464.64	0.57	NS
Interaction	0.09	1	0.09	0.00	NS
Error	–	∞	820.70	–	–

* Incidence of rehospitalization.

Competence Scale and posthospital outcome among psychiatric patients. However, the finding that this relationship holds only for schizophrenic patients, and can be entirely attributed to the age the patient first entered psychiatric treatment, seriously questions the construct validity of the above scale as a measure of premorbid social competence, as well as its adequacy in testing the developmental approach advocated by Zigler and Phillips.[3, 5]

Any attempt to devise a performance scale applicable to all age levels must ensure that a subject's score on each of the component variables is solely dependent upon age, appropriate ability, or performance. The Zigler and Phillips' Social Competence Scale does not meet this criterion. In addition, the possibility raised earlier that the scale might be an appropriate prognostic indicator among adult patients only was not supported by our data. The results of this study indicate that the prognostic value of the Zigler and Phillips' Social Competence Scale seems to be completely an epiphenomenon of age at first psychiatric treatment contact.

This finding emphasizes the problems involved in attempting to interpret results on the basis of the face validity of a predictive scale, and points out the need for the application of more stringent statistical procedures in the construction and reporting of prognostic scales. Specifically, had data relating to the criterion validity of the items, as well as the internal consistency of the scale, been reported originally, the present findings should have been self-evident. That this problem is not unique to Zigler and Phillips is indicated by the results of other investigations,[12, 13] which suggest that the prognostic value of three widely used multi-item scales (the Elgin, the Kantor, and the Phillips scales) is due to their relationship with marital status.

Although the present study raises some important methodologic issues regarding the validity of the Zigler and Phillips Scale as a measure of premorbid social competence, it does not necessarily refute the possible importance of the premorbid social competence construct as a prognostic indicator among psychiatric patients. The explanation has been offered,[14] in line with Zigler and Phillips' theoretic approach, that the later the onset of illness, as estimated by the patient's age at first psychiatric treatment contact, the later the patient's development of competence is interrupted. Therefore a higher level of social competence should be attained and the patient should have a greater ability to cope successfully once more with the expectations of society. It is the level of premorbid competence that sets the limit of competence to which a patient can return during remission. Definitions of social competence appropriate to each age level must still be developed, in order to adequately test the prognostic utility of the premorbid social competence construct.

The results of this study emphasize the need for taking into account the age the patient first entered psychiatric treatment in determining the appropriate definition of premorbid social competence for the specific patient. Once this has been done, it should then be possible to determine whether, in fact, premorbid social competence is related to prognosis.

The lack of a significant relationship between incidence of re-hospitalization and either social competence or age at first psychiatric treatment contact for nonschizophrenic patients further questions Zigler and Phillips'[3, 5] unitary theory of psychopathology. It also demonstrates that age at first treatment is not a unitary phenomenon, but has an interactive significance derived from diagnosis.

Although the present discussion deals specifically with the relationship between social competence and prognosis, there have been attempts to extend this explanation to imply causal relationships between social competence and the incidence of mental illness,[3] type of symptom,[5] as well as the process of entering a schizophrenic episode.[14] This point of view ignores the possibility that social competence itself may be the end result of a variety of biologic and psychologic as well as social factors. For instance, the hypothesis can be raised that the occurrence of schizophrenia early in life reflects a basic limitation of the patient's central nervous system (CNS), which in turn limits the patient's ability to develop a higher level of premorbid competence.

It is the burden of our argument that seemingly unitary phenomena, such as social competence, or age at first psychiatric treatment contact, reflect a diversity of processes. To study mental disorder, a more refined analysis that includes the exploration of biologic, diagnostic, and psychologic as well as social factors is necessary.

SUMMARY

The three-year posthospital outcome of a group of 166 previously hospitalized psychiatric patients was determined. A significant relationship was found between the incidence of rehospitalization and both age at first psychiatric treatment contact ($P<0.001$) and Zigler and Phillips' Social Competence Scale ($P<0.001$). However, the two predictor variables were significantly related ($\phi = 0.71$, $P<0.001$), and the prognostic value of the Zigler and Phillips Scale was based entirely upon its relationship with age at first psychiatric treatment contact. Further, its value was limited to schizophrenic patients, thus indicating that the meanings of both age at first treatment contact and social competence were functions of diagnosis rather than panpsychopathologic indexes. The need for developing age-appropriate definitions of social competence was discussed.

REFERENCES

1. Levenstein, S., Klein, D. F., and Pollack, M.: Follow-Up Study of Formerly Hospitalized Voluntary Psychiatric Patients: First Two Years, *Amer. J. Psychiat.*, 122:1102–1109, April 1966.
2. Pollack, M., Levenstein, S., and Klein, D. F.: Three-Year Posthospital Follow-Up of Adolescent and Adult Schizophrenics, *Amer. J. Orthopsychiat.*, 38:94–109, January 1968.

3. Zigler, E., and Phillips, L.: Social Competence and Outcome in Psychiatric Disorder, *J. Abnorm. Soc. Psychol.*, 63:264–271, August 1961.
4. Phillips, L.: "Social Competence, Process-Reactive Distinction and Nature of Mental Disorder," in Hoch, P. H., and Zubin, J. (eds.): *Psychopathology of Schizophrenia*, New York: Grune & Stratton, 1966, pp. 471–481.
5. Zigler, E., and Phillips, L.: Social Competence and Process-Reactive Distinction in Psychopathology, *J. Abnorm. Psychol.*, 65:215–222, October 1962.
6. Dorland, W. A.: *American Medical Dictionary*, Philadelphia: W. B. Saunders, 1948, p. 1172.
7. Levenstein, S., Pollack, M., and Klein, D. F.: Follow-up Study of Formerly Hospitalized Voluntary Psychiatric Patients: Considerations in Data Collection, *J. Hillside Hospital*, 15:152–164, July–October 1966.
8. Klein, D. F.: Importance of Psychiatric Diagnosis in Prediction of Clinical Drug Effects, *Arch. Gen. Psychiat.*, 16:118–126, January 1967.
9. Rao, C. R.: *Linear Statistical Inference and Its Applications*, New York: John Wiley & Sons, 1965, pp. 358–362.
10. Snedecor, G. W.: *Statistical Methods*, ed. 5, Ames, Iowa: Iowa State University Press, 1956, pp. 231, 338, 380, 384.
11. Rosen, B., et al: Social Competence and Posthospital Outcome Among Schizophrenic and Nonschizophrenic Psychiatric Patients, *J. Abnorm. Psychiat.* To be published.
12. Chapman, L. J., Day, D., and Burstein, A.: Process-Reactive Distinction and Prognosis in Schizophrenia, *J. Nerv. Ment. Dis.*, 133:383–391, April 1961.
13. Garfield, S. L., and Sundland, D. M.: Prognostic Scales in Schizophrenia, *J. Consult. Psychol.*, 30:13–24.
14. National Institute of Mental Health, Psychopharmacology Research Branch Collaborative Study Group: Short-Term Improvement in Schizophrenia: Contribution of Background Factors, *Amer. J. Psychiat.*, 124:900–909, January 1968.

14

Changing Perspectives
in Research and the Treatment
of the Schizophrenic Patient*

by PHILIP R. A. MAY

May discusses the difficulties and travail of a research team in a mental hospital. He delineates the interpersonal problems related to administering research and overcoming disharmonious relationships during an experiment. We are shown how carefully planned and designed experiments can be ruined unless skill is applied to integrate the mental hospital staff with the research team. May then summarizes the results of his study on schizophrenia. With 228 schizophrenic patients treated with tranquilizing drugs—alone, or combined with psychotherapy—proof is offered that such treatment may have been the most effective and efficient for the largest percentage of this group of schizophrenic patients. Individual psychotherapy and milieu therapy alone were found to be the least effective, most expensive, and most time-consuming. Electroconvulsive therapy was rated between two extremes.

This chapter emphasizes that training in treatment flexibility must be spread to the total psychiatric staff, that a closed mind in psychiatry is a detriment to research and treatment. The flexible attitude in psychiatry is

* This paper originates in part from the Schizophrenia Research Project supported by the Psychopharmacology Service Center, NIMH, USPHS. Contract PH 43 66 49; research grants NIMH 02719 and NIMH 04589; grants from the State of California, Department of Mental Hygiene as well as from the Albert A. Epstein Fund of the Rush Research Foundation, Los Angeles, California.

a valuable tool for research and clinical treatment and, as he points out, should be part of the initial training of every psychiatrist.

Psychiatric research presently attracts a great deal of attention, but its ultimate role must be viewed in perspective and its results interpreted in terms of patient care and professional education. To some, research represents the noble knight prepared to deliver the Holy Grail; to others, it is merely the acquisition of facts that have little practical use. The purpose of this chapter is to discuss clinical psychiatric research as a function that must be integrated realistically into teaching and patient care, using as an illustration the author's research interest—the schizophrenic patient.

Perhaps the first point that should be made is that the integration of clinical research into the other functions of an institution is not just a matter of applying results attained by others. Passive receptivity is not enough. Simple cooperation is not enough. We must create an atmosphere in which the research investigator *and the entire institution* have a sense of active participation in a commonly shared and important experience—the improvement of patient care.

Whatever the psychiatric setting, a clinical research project will be successful only if the investigator has some understanding of the institution and its operation, as well as a cohesive working relationship with its staff. He must be fully aware of the kind of transactions, bypaths, and inefficiencies that might ruin his design or contaminate his data, and must be prepared to handle such difficulties positively and effectively, yet with consideration and an understanding of the underlying personal human factors that can mitigate against successful research.

The most searching design for the evaluation of treatment of schizophrenia falls to pieces if, for example, the investigator lacks sufficient know-how to prevent dropouts. The research design also can be adversely affected if he fails to recognize that a rigidly timed schedule of treatment or testing could conflict with visitors, attendance at baseball games, work therapy, and other realities of hospital life. If a research design for the evaluation of psychotherapy ignores the fact that schizophrenic patients are likely to be given antipsychotic drugs, it can hardly be called realistic. And any research experiment will prove worthless and unreliable if the investigator is unable to gain the *effective* (as opposed to the *nominal*) cooperation of the treating physicians.

Little confidence can be placed in data obtained from routine hospital records, or from rating scales disseminated to busy and hardworking staff by whom the investigator may be considered, at best, a nuisance. It requires more than pledges of mutual goodwill and cooperation, more than ivory-tower theorizing, to execute a research design effectively in an institutional setting. What it takes is a particular kind of administrative and interpersonal skill, plus the ability to cope with unpredictable obstructions. If these qualities are lacking, errors can all too easily occur and be compounded under the charisma of research. Such errors do occur all too frequently, but are rarely discussed, of course, in a research project.

The positive aspect of having these qualities was illustrated very clearly to me a few years ago when I visited a number of different hospitals that were cooperating in a collaborative research project. The superintendent of one of these hospitals was the investigator in charge; participating vigorously, enthusiastically, and effectively, he was conspicuously free from complaints of inefficiency and lack of cooperation. His research staff was proud of the efficiency with which they were able to execute the research design. Hardly surprising? Perhaps. But the question is: How many textbooks of experimental design contain a chapter on practical research administration? How many even mention that it helps to be on good terms with the superintendent of nurses, the head nurse, and the medical staff? How many of the pundits who thunder about the virtues of reliability attempt to distinguish between the reliability of an experiment (ie, reliability of execution of project design) and the reliability of a test instrument?

I would agree completely with those hospital superintendents and chiefs of research who insist that any research project conducted in their institution by an outside investigator should have at least one active participant from the staff of the institution. It is worthwhile for the outside investigator to train a staff man from scratch if necessary. Indeed, the sophisticated outside investigator would not dream of attempting a project otherwise, for he knows that the reliability of his project can depend to a large degree on having such a participant.

The integration of research should begin very early, a research attitude being inculcated in the course of professional training. The climate of medical care is changing swiftly from art to science. Not so long ago a physician could practice all his life, usually without a great deal of change, the techniques of diagnosis and treatment that had been passed along to him by his predecessors. The style of psychiatric education was then essentially that of an apprentice learning his profession from skilled and worthy masters.

This has changed, and it is to be doubted that psychiatry can afford to linger in its present stage; styles and techniques of psychiatric practice are also likely to change one or two generations from now. It would seem preferable, therefore, to teach our residents, interns, and students to adopt a flexible research attitude. They should become aware of the numerous directions in which psychiatric research is moving; they should adopt the attitude that since change is inevitable, the task is to guide the process in a positive direction, to question, and to strive for precision always, to define the borderline between fact and opinion, between legitimate conclusions and mere speculation. At the same time, they should accept the reality that there are great inadequacies and gaps in the present state of psychiatric art and science, and that decisions as to the care of the individual patient often have to be made on the basis of opinion. They must always be open to new speculations or alternative hypotheses, avoiding old or new dogmas.

It would be unfortunate—and erroneous—to equate science or research with laboratory procedures. Feinstein, in an excellent series of articles,[1-4] has illustrated the thesis that the clinician is a measuring instrument in his own right, and that a research attitude can be applied to clinical data and procedures as well as to those of the laboratory. The one cannot substitute for the other, however, and our education should communicate the fact that in their different but complementary ways both the laboratory and the clinician can contribute to the progress of medical science.

Hopefully, our education also would invalidate the need to refute the belief of Max Planck[5] that "a new scientific truth does not triumph by convincing its opponents and making them see the light, but rather because its opponents eventually die, and a new generation grows up that is familiar with it." Our flexible educators must present to the neophyte all the latest research data, even though it may contradict their own biases.

In this context, it is of interest to consider the practical implications that might be drawn from some of the more recent research studies of the treatment of schizophrenia, to ascertain to what extent these run counter to the resistances of well-worn belief or to the fashion of the moment. In the 1940s and 1950s it was the practice, in some circles, to treat the schizophrenic by settling him down into a comfortable form of therapeutic hospital milieu with a nice blend of activity, humanitarianism, democratic process, individual therapy, and group interaction among the patients and staff. All that was needed, it seemed, was more and more staff and a more and more therapeutic hospital milieu. The advent of antipsychotic drugs and the associated wave of research have changed all this. Experimental evidence from controlled research studies indicates that when the powerful effect of antipsychotic drugs is considered, the results of hospital treatment are equally good at all levels of milieu care, except under circumstances of virtual neglect or gross deficiency. Should we not, then, perhaps redirect our staff time and effort from improving the hospital milieu to helping our patients stay out of the hospital? With drugs, not only can we help them stay out; we also can help more patients out of hospitals more quickly and without any loss in quality of result.

To illustrate this point by reference to actual research studies, Greenblatt, Solomon, Evans, and Brooks[6] selected chronic schizophrenic patients from the population of two state hospitals and divided them into four groups. The patients in two of the groups remained at the parent state hospitals, one receiving drugs, the other no drugs. The remainder were transferred to the Massachusetts Mental Health Center, half on drug therapy and half receiving no drug therapy. Thus, the study evaluated drug therapy at two levels of care: (1) routine "custodial," and (2) a highly active, intensive treatment program in a research, training, and intensive treatment center.

Their main finding was that antipsychotic drugs produced significant clinical improvement compared with the controls. This finding manifested itself irrespective of widely disparate clinical settings. The intensive active milieu by itself failed to produce significant improvement during the same period of time. Though there were more discharges from the active milieu (with and without drug), this was attributed to a very active social service department and the availability of day-hospital facilities, suggesting that the main effect of the active milieu was confined to better discharge planning. (In follow-up, there was some suggestion that there might have been a delayed beneficial effect from the active program. This part of the study was uncontrolled, and one cannot be certain whether to attribute the further improvement in these patients to continued drug therapy or to the aftereffects of the milieu, or to both.)

In a five-year follow-up by Letemendia, Harris, and Willems,[7] no striking changes in mental state were found to accompany either the introduction of an open ward policy or of treatment in a "therapeutic community." (There was actually some improvement in occupation as well as some deterioration in personal habits, both more marked in the "therapeutic community" than in the other division of the hospital.) The investigators conclude that "as far as the long-stay schizophrenic patients are concerned, the case for the adoption of 'therapeutic community' measures must rest on general humanitarian grounds, rather than on the therapeutic benefit to be derived."

Humdziak and Pasamanick[8] also question seriously whether it is at present justifiable to invest much time and effort in hospital activity programs. In their study, three groups of patients were assigned respectively to regular occupational therapy, intensive occupational therapy, and industrial therapy, and a fourth group, a control group, was specifically excluded from any occupational or industrial therapy. The three activity groups were always rated as more improved than the controls, with regular O.T. (not intensive) usually the highest. The differences were not statistically significant, and the investigators felt these could be accounted for by bias on the part of the raters rather than by any true differences in the program effects.

Evangelakis[9] found that drugs were effective at all levels of care, to such an extent that better results were obtained *with* drug in a minimal custody setting than *without* drug in a setting of intensive care. The addition of intensive care to drug therapy did improve the results further, up to a point. The results were better in the two highest levels of care than in minimal custody, but equal at these two levels.

Appleby[10] found no significant differences among three different levels of intensive care. In fact, those assigned to a special program designed to maximize interpersonal therapeutic clarity and effectiveness improved more slowly than the others, whereas the patients assigned to more conventional programs showed significantly less perceptual distortion and less paranoid thinking. However, the special-program patients did achieve a better balance on submissiveness and hostility.

Honigfeld, et al,[11] in a group program found no significant evidence of enhancement of drug effect in older chronic schizophrenic patients. (Interestingly, group therapy did seem to enhance the effect of placebo.)

Hamilton, et al,[12] observed a difference between the sexes, somewhat hard to interpret. In females, the results—and the drug advantage—were the same for intensive treatment and routine milieu care. In males, intensive treatment had an effect significantly greater than routine care and roughly comparable to that of drugs. In the latter there also was evidence of a ceiling effect: either drugs or intensive milieu care seemed to improve these patients to a point beyond which the addition of the other method caused little difference. Thus a moderate drug effect could be enhanced by intensive milieu care, but not render the effect of a powerful drug.

In a study by Cooper[13] one group of schizophrenic patients was treated with antipsychotic drugs without any organized program of activity, and another received no drugs but had a carefully organized milieu program of intensive group activities and individual attention. At the end of 24 weeks the drug group (without any activity program) had improved more than the intensive activity group, though not significantly so.

The findings of the studies reviewed above do not contradict those of our own Schizophrenia Research Project[14]—that drug therapy produced major benefit when enriched with a milieu that could be considered reasonably attainable in a public hospital.

The NIMH Psychopharmacology Service Center Collaborative Group[15] found that the amount of placebo-drug differences did not vary significantly, whatever the hospital setting. In brief, the majority of research relative to these projects showed that the drug was the significant factor compared to the milieu.

It would be well to keep in mind Cole's comment[16] that a toxic dose of environmental stimulation is conceivable, just as is a toxic dose of drugs. It is certainly possible that both a barren custodial milieu and an overactive one could be deleterious to schizophrenic patients with limited psychic resources.

In the area of alternatives to hospital treatment for the schizophrenic patient, it is proposed that we also preserve a flexible research attitude. The current trend toward community maintenance for the schizophrenic patient has been long overdue, but it would be advisable to ask for a controlled study of the financial and personal cost of the various intra- and extramural programs before making any overly optimistic decision in this particular matter. The studies of Grad and Sainsbury,[17,18] and Hogarty, et al,[19] imply that we treat with reserve some of the therapeutic claims for various "community" programs.

Here again, as in the case of in-hospital milieu, there may be a ceiling effect. Possibly more is to be gained by developing specific treatment methods than by raising the level of "nonspecific" social care above a certain point. Adequately controlled studies of different levels of community care are not available at the moment; however, antipsychotic drugs have been reported to be effective even in the context of a good level of community care: eg, Charalampous;[20] Dinitz, et al;[21] Pasamanick, et al;[22] Scarpitti, et al;[23] and Kris.[24-26]

Controlled research also would indicate that, in general, little is to be gained by directing resources toward providing psychotherapy for the schizophrenic patient while he is in the hospital. Grinspoon, Ewalt, and Shader[27] found that patients treated in the hospital solely, by well-qualified therapists with intensive individual psychotherapy, did not appear to change over the course of two years. However, by comparison, there was statistically significant improvement in patients treated with the combination of drug and psychotherapy. The investigators comment that their findings do not bear out the claim of some psychotherapists that pharmacotherapy interferes with progress in psychotherapy.

Reports on the first 100 patients in our own Schizophrenia Research Project[28,29] indicated no significant difference between drug alone and psychotherapy plus drug in terms of the following: release rate; length of hospital stay and amount of time in the hospital during the first three years after admission; amount of sedatives and hydrotherapy required; change in overall status as judged by psychoanalysts; and ratings of final status by nurses and psychoanalysts. Nor was there any difference in readmission rates. These findings are now supported by more detailed analyses covering an extensive number of criteria on 228 patients,[14] which indicate that for the immediate outcome of hospital treatment, the differences between drug alone and drug plus psychotherapy were mainly small and insubstantial and never impressive. Moreover, such interaction as did occur between the two forms of treatment was mainly in the direction of potentiation of a positive drug effect on certain variables where psychotherapy alone, given in the hospital, appeared to have little effect or even a slightly adverse effect.

It is to be emphasized that such a finding as related to the treatment of hospitalized schizophrenic patients should not lead us to conclude that research studies advise us to neglect their psychological needs. As I have commented elsewhere,[14] a distinction needs to be made between *psychotherapy* and *what is therapeutic for the psyche;* between *psychotherapy* and *psychotherapeutic management;* and between the *inpatient* and the *outpatient* phases of treatment. In my opinion, an optimal level of *psychotherapeutic management* (which may include laying the groundwork for formal psychotherapy) is highly desirable in the treatment of the schizophrenic patient, both in and out of the hospital. *Formal psychotherapy,* on the other hand, would seem to have its main indication in the outpatient phase, after restitution has been achieved and when the need is for stabilization of the personality.

It is also important to consider that psychotherapy may have a potential role to play in the hospital treatment of those patients who fail to respond to drug therapy. I have remarked elsewhere[14] that if there are indeed patients who respond specifically to psychotherapy, they are likely to be concentrated in the group who have failed to respond to drug therapy. Moreover, it is precisely this group of failure patients that would seem to be deserving of our maximum psychotherapeutic efforts.

This brings me to a concluding comment on the subject of integrating research into the treatment function of a hospital. The comparative financial cost figures developed by our Schizophrenia Research Project[14] and the controlled studies referred to elsewhere in this chapter lead this author to question most seriously and deeply the financial and therapeutic wisdom of the prevalent dogma of allocation of resources for hospital treatment. It is a dogma that provides the highest level of care for newly admitted cases and transfers the failures of this initial period of "intensive treatment" to less well-staffed units or hospitals. I would suggest that the results of our research indicate the procedure be somewhat different—ie, transfer the *failures* to a special multidisciplinary treatment research unit staffed at a *higher* level and with *better* facilities than the rest of the hospital. Such a research unit should be able to provide as necessary and desirable, in a controlled research setting, any form of treatment, including the most recent developments. This would be one way to integrate our research and treatment resources into an obvious working partnership and direct them toward an area of maximum need and greatest suffering.

SUMMARY

Clinical psychiatric research is a function that should be integrated realistically into teaching and patient care. It should not be just a matter of the mere passive application of the results of others. It should start with a professional training that accepts change as an active, constructive, participant process, and so inculcates a flexible research attitude. In the institution, clinical research requires also a degree of administrative expertise on the part of the research investigator.

Research studies on the treatment of schizophrenia are reviewed. The demonstrable value of drug treatment is emphasized. The exaggerated use of intensive psychotherapy is elucidated. The suggestion is made that different subtypes of schizophrenic patients may be responsive to special treatment programs.

REFERENCES

1. Feinstein, A. R.: Scientific Methodology in Clinical Medicine: I. Introduction, Principles, and Concepts, *Ann. Intern. Med.*, 61:564–579, 1964.
2. Feinstein, A. R.: Scientific Methodology in Clinical Medicine: II. Classification of Human Disease by Clinical Behavior, *Ann. Intern. Med.*, 61:757–781, 1964.
3. Feinstein, A. R.: Scientific Methodology in Clinical Medicine: III. The Evaluation of Therapeutic Response, *Ann. Intern. Med.*, 61:944–965, 1964.
4. Feinstein, A. R.: Scientific Methodology in Clinical Medicine: IV. Acquisition of Clinical Data, *Ann. Intern. Med.*, 61:1162–1193, 1964.
5. Planck, M.: *Scientific Autobiography and Other Papers,* New York: Philosophical Library, 1949, pp. 33–34.
6. Greenblatt, M., Solomon, M. H., Evans, A. S., and Brooks, G. W. (eds.): *Drug and Social Therapy in Chronic Schizophrenia,* Springfield, Ill.: Charles C. Thomas, 1965.
7. Letemendia, F. J. J., Harris, A. D., and Willems, P. J. A.: Clinical Effects on Population of Chronic Schizophrenic Patients of Administrative Changes in Hospital, *Brit. J. Psychiat.*, 113:959–971, 1967.
8. Humdziak, M., and Pasamanick, B.: Occupational and Industrial Therapy in Treatment of Psychiatric Patients: Controlled Study of Efficacy in Intensive Treatment Institution, *Genet. Psycholog. Monogr.*, 69:3–48, 1964.
9. Evangelakis, M. D.: De-institutionalization of Patients (Triad of Trifluoperazine-Group Psychotherapy-Adjunctive Therapy), *Dis. Nerv. Syst.*, 22:26–32, 1961.
10. Appleby, L.: Evaluation of Treatment Methods for Chronic Schizophrenia, *Arch. Gen. Psychiat.*, 8:8–21, 1963.
11. Honigfeld, G., Rosenblum, M. P., Blumenthal, I. J., Lambert, H. L., and Roberts, A. J.: Behavioral Improvement in Older Schizophrenic Patient: Drug and Social Therapies, *J. Amer. Geriat. Soc.*, 13:57–72, 1965.
12. Hamilton, M., Hordern, A., Waldrop, F. N., and Lofft, J.: Controlled Trial on Value of Prochlorperazine, Trifluoperazine and Intensive Group Treatment, *Brit. J. Psychiat.*, 109:510–522, 1963.

13. Cooper, B.: Grouping and Tranquilizers in Chronic Ward, *Brit. J. Med. Psychol.*, 34:157–162, 1961.
14. May, P. R. A.: *Treatment of Schizophrenia: Comparative Study of Five Treatment Methods*, New York: Science House, 1968.
15. Goldberg, S. C.: Personal communication.
16. Cole, J. O.: Lack of Controls, *Int. J. Psychiat.*, 4:129–131, **1967.**
17. Grad, J. C., and Sainsbury, P.: Mental Illness and The Family, *Lancet*, 1:544–547, 1963.
18. Grad, J. C., and Sainsbury, P.: Problems of Caring for Mentally Ill at Home, *Proc. Roy. Soc. Med.*, 59:20–23, 1966.
19. Hogarty, G. E., Dennis, H., Guy, W., and Gross, G. M.: Who Goes There?: Critical Evaluation of Admission to Day Hospital, *Amer. J. Psychiat.*, 124: 934–944, 1968.
20. Charalampous, K. D. (ed.): Long-Term Care of Chronic Mentally Ill Patient: Medical Approach, *Medical Record and Annals*, 56:257–258, 1963.
21. Dinitz, S., Scarpitti, F. R., Albini, J. L., Lefton, M., and Pasamanick, B.: Experimental Study in the Prevention of Hospitalization of Schizophrenics, *Amer. J. Orthopsychiat.*, 35(1):1–9, 1965.
22. Pasamanick, B., Scarpitti, F. R., Lefton, M., Dinitz, S., Wernert, J. J., and McPheeters, H.: Home vs Hospital Care for Schizophrenics, *JAMA*, 187: 177–181, 1964.
23. Scarpitti, F. R., Lefton, M., Dinitz, S., and Pasamanick, B.: Problems in Home-Care Study for Schizophrenics, *Arch. Gen. Psychiat.*, 10:143–154, 1964.
24. Kris, E. B.: Aftercare and Rehabilitation of Mentally Ill, *Curr. Ther. Res.*, 5:24–30, 1963.
25. Kris, E. B.: Five-Year Community Follow-up of Patients Discharged from a Mental Hospital, *Curr. Ther. Res.*, 5:451–462, 1963.
26. Kris, E. B.: Five Years Experience with Use of Drug and Psychotherapy in Community Aftercare Clinic, *Amer. J. Public Health*, 52(suppl.):9–12, 1962.
27. Grinspoon, L., Ewalt, J. R., and Shader, R.: Long Term Treatment of Chronic Schizophrenia: Preliminary Report, *Int. J. Psychiat.*, 4:116–128, 1967.
28. May, P. R. A., and Tuma, A. H.: Ataraxic Drugs and Psychotherapy: Effect of Psychotherapy and Stelazine on Length of Hospital Stay, Release Rate, and Supplemental Treatment of Schizophrenic Patients, *J. Nerv. Ment. Dis.*, 139:362–369, 1964.
29. May, P. R. A., and Tuma, A. H.: Treatment of Schizophrenia, *Brit. J. Psychiat.*, 3:503–510, 1965.

15

The Need for Extensive Reform in Psychiatric Teaching: An Investigation in Treatment Ideology and Learning*

by CHING-PIAO CHIEN†
and WILLIAM S. APPLETON

This study raises important questions concerning the education of psychiatric residents. Chien shows that when our own beliefs become a deep unconscious bias in practicing psychopharmacology, we are unable to learn and accept new data without distortion. Chien urges greater flexibility in psychiatric teaching and practice. He stimulates us to reformulate our previous teaching methods and shows, by his own clear use of the scientific method, how to be aware of our rigidities; he clarifies the injuries that our deeply held and previously accepted false speculations may produce. This chapter demonstrates that our manner of educating psychiatrists needs important changes.

* This study was done at the Massachusetts Mental Health Center under grant FR 055504 from General Research Support.

The authors gratefully acknowledge the help and advice given by Drs. Jack Ewalt, Gerald Klerman, Myron Sharaf, Alberto DiMascio, and Mrs. Evelyn M. Stone.

† This study was done when the senior author was a Teaching Fellow in Psychiatry, Harvard Medical School, at the Massachusetts Mental Health Center.

The rapid growth of psychopharmacology during the past decade has been stimulated by the therapeutic success of chlorpromazine (Thorazine), reserpine, and meprobamate (MILTOWN/ EQUANIL). Research in this field ranges from the biochemical approach in laboratories to behavioral studies in mental hospitals. Of the hundreds of compounds evaluated, over two dozen have been approved by the Food and Drug Administration for therapeutic use. The pragmatic role of drug therapy in present-day psychiatry is so undeniable that attempts have even been made to integrate drugs within the framework of psychodynamic concepts.[1-4]

Despite the importance of drug therapy, and in contrast to the progress that has been made in recent years in the understanding and use of psychotropic drugs, little attention has been given to evaluating the methods employed and problems encountered in the teaching of psychopharmacology.[5] Recently, several psychiatric educators have pointed out the need for more thorough supervision of residents in this field.[6-8]

Many authors have shown that the psychodynamic approach is predominant in American psychiatry, particularly among residents primarily interested in preparation for private practice.[9, 10] The *American Handbook of Psychiatry* states: "At the present time, the majority of residents are most interested in psychodynamic psychiatry and particularly in psychoanalysis."[11] In contrasting the prestige and emphasis on dynamic psychotherapy, drug treatment was reported as "uncared for" and "second class" in American psychiatry.[12] Klerman[6] stated that "psychopharmacology is regarded by many residents as of low priority and by some residents as extraneous to the main goals of their training." Freyhan[7] pointed out that "first-year residents are often given what amounts to a free hand when it comes to drug treatment while systematic supervision is—rightfully—considered an absolute necessity for psychotherapy."

RATIONALE OF PRESENT STUDY

There is little argument that the psychiatric resident's use of drugs is inadequately supervised. This lack is particularly due to the fact that drug therapy is a relatively new field and also to the fact that ideologic emphasis is on psychotherapy. The psychotherapeutically oriented resident is likely to be less motivated to learn psychopharmacology than his eclectic colleague. This difference in motivation and the consequent acquisition of knowledge may be even greater when systematic and compulsory instruction in psychopharmacology is not a part of the resident's first-year training. But when it is, what situation results—to what extent does ideology influence the physician's learning of drug treatment; how is drug practice related to the resident's ideology?

The Massachusetts Mental Health Center study was undertaken in an effort to answer these questions. Also, the teaching program in psychopharmacology provided at this university hospital was examined to see how effective it was, what improvements might be made, and what others might learn from our experience.

LOCALE OF STUDY AND TRAINING PROGRAM

The Massachusetts Mental Health Center is a Harvard University Medical School psychiatric teaching, treatment, and research center in which 70 psychiatric residents and fellows are in training. Twenty-four of these are first-year residents assigned to the inpatient services. Many members of the senior staff are psychoanalysts. Psychodynamic theory and training in psychotherapy are major focuses of the residency program. Emphasis is also placed on social and community psychiatry. The social structure and milieu of the wards are being reevaluated continually.[13-18]

Although psychotherapy is the most highly valued method of treatment, a large proportion of the patients, especially on the inpatient services, receive some form of somatic therapy. From 40% to 60% of patients admitted since 1954 have received drugs.[17-22] This percentage has shown a moderate increase over the past decade.

Because of the importance of drugs and the frequency with which they are used, a psychopharmacologic training program for first-year residents was established about ten years ago to:

1. Teach the therapeutic uses, the physiologic biochemistry, the pharmacologic actions, the contraindications, and the side effects of the various psychoactive agents.

2. Provide an understanding of the social and psychologic aspects of drugs in the total treatment program, especially psychotherapy.

3. Stimulate systematic observation in this area and encourage the careful evaluation of research claims.

A psychopharmacology seminar is held once a week for a six-month period during the first year of residency training. The topics include the physiologic, biochemical, and pharmacologic actions of the various agents, and the principles of evaluation of treatment. The seminar usually consists of four parts: (1) special modalities and problems of treatment; (2) cellular mechanism of drug action (biochemical aspect); (3) cellular mechanism of drug action (bio-electric aspect); and (4) psychobiologic mechanism of drug action.

One-hour walking rounds for first-year residents are conducted by the chief of the drug unit twice weekly on the inpatient services. Treatment indications, dosage, and the management of side effects are reviewed in the context of individual patients and their clinical needs. Each first-year resident is associated with the drug unit for a two-month rotation, at which time he participates in rounds and serves as liaison between his service unit and the drug therapy group. Continual consultation and liaison between ward staff and psychopharmacology experts is thereby provided. In addition, a full-time special attendant observes patients daily for therapeutic and side effects, keeps records of drug use, and presents problem cases during teaching rounds. He thus serves as an important liaison between the residents and the drug unit.

PROCEDURE

A group of 24 physicians, all just beginning their psychiatric residency, were used as the subjects of this investigation. The Mason and Sachs Chemotherapy Attitude Questionnaire[23] and a psychopharmacologic knowledge questionnaire—hereafter called Drug Knowledge Test—were administered during the first week of residency. The same attitude and knowledge questionnaires were readministered six months later when the systematic course in psychopharmacology had been completed.

The residents were divided into psychotherapeutic and eclectic groups on the basis of Factor E of the aforementioned Mason and Sachs Chemotherapy Attitude Scale.[23] Factor E is an index of ideology with respect to drugs versus psychotherapy. The statements comprising this factor are (1) Drugs substitute artificial controls for real ego-strengthening; (2) The best way to help a patient is by increasing self-understanding through psychotherapy; and (3) Improvement through psychotherapy tends to be more genuine and longer-lasting than can be achieved through drug therapy. Each statement is scored on a five-point scale, ranging from "strongly agree" ($+2$) to "strongly disagree" (-2). Thus, the sum of the scores ranges from +6 to −6. We assume that those residents whose total score is on the plus side (+1 to +6) regard psychotherapy as a superior form of treatment, and they therefore are classified as *psychotherapeutic;* those whose total score equals zero or a minus number (0 to −6) are considered to be uncertain, or opposed to this view, and we have labeled them *eclectic*.

The Drug Knowledge Test* was constructed specifically for our study; it contains 28 major questions with 123 items from which 106 correct answers can be drawn. The maximal score on this test is therefore 106. Since the range of psychopharmacology is so wide, we tried to select questions that relate closely to clinical priactice. Emphasis was placed especially on the knowledge of side effects. The 106 items can be grouped under five different aspects of knowledge about psychopharmacology. (Three of these items overlap, making the total number of items 109.) They are:

1. Side Effects (65 items)
   eg *Question 6*. In the following list, check chlorpromazine (Thorazine) side effects: (1) jaundice; (2) neuritis; (3) parkinsonism; (4) vitamin B deficiency; (5) blood dyscrasia; (6) skin rash; [and so on up to] (23) lenticular opacities.
2. Classification (18 items)
   eg *Question 18*. Check the drug that belongs to the MAO inhibitor class: (1) promazine (Sparine); (2) diazepam (Valium); (3) isocarboxazid (Marplan); (4) amitriptyline HCl (Elavil); (5) nialamide (Niamid); (6) chlordiazepoxide (Librium); (7) benactyzine HCl (Deprol).
3. Indications and Contraindications (10 items)
   eg *Question 27*. Generally speaking, some of the following are considered as contraindications for phenothiazine treatment. Please check those which are contraindications: (1) comatose state; (2) liver disease; (3) status epilepticus; (4) barbiturate overdosage; (5) morning sickness.
4. Effectiveness and Dosage (7 items)
   eg *Question 9*. For schizophrenics, long term medication frequently prevents rehospitalization. True____ False____.

* More than 200 questions were prepared by the authors as a first step. This initial questionnaire was then sent out to four hospital staff members active in psychopharmacology. The answers of the staff members were compared, and 106 test items were selected on the basis of the consistency of the staff responses. After six months the authors were tested again; the answers remained up to 98% consistent with their original responses, thereby indicating that the questionnaire had retained its validity during the six-month period despite new developments in the field.

5. Psychosocial Factors in Drug Treatment (9 items)

eg *Question 11.* The main effect of a phenothiazine is achieved through the doctor's attitude in giving it. True_____ False_____.

RESULTS

1. *Initial Ideology Related to Initial Amount of Psychopharmaco-logic Knowledge*

At the beginning of their psychiatric careers, there were 16 residents in the psychotherapeutic category and eight classified as eclectic. The total mean of these 24 first-year residents' psychopharmacologic knowledge score was 65.7 (62% right answers on the Drug Knowledge Test). The mean score for the psychotherapeutic residents was 63.5; for the eclectic resident it was 68.7. This difference is not statistically significant. It is interesting to note that although these first-year residents began their psychiatric career with different treatment ideologies, there did not appear to be any significant difference in the total amount of psychopharmacologic knowledge they had absorbed prior to their residency.

TABLE 1

Initial Ideology Related to Initial Amount of Psychopharmacologic Knowledge

	Psychotherapeutic	Eclectic	Total
Number of residents	16	8	24
Mean score of psycho-pharmacologic knowledge	63.5*	68.7*	65.7

* Difference between "psychotherapeutic" and "eclectic" groups is not significant: t = 1.26, d.f. = 22, P > 0.1.

2. *Ideology Related to Amount of Psychopharmacologic Knowledge After a Six-Month Training Program*

On retesting, after a six-month training program, the mean score for all on the Drug Knowledge Test was 82.6 (78% right answers). At the end of six months, four of the originally psychotherapeutic residents shifted into the eclectic group, whereas two residents changed from eclectic to psychotherapeutic. There was thus a 25%

change within each group. The difference btween the two groups in terms of changing ideology is not significant, as shown in Table 2.

TABLE 2
Change of Ideology of First-Year Resident

		AFTER SIX MONTHS	
		Eclectic	Psychotherapeutic
Beginning	Psychotherapeutic	4	12
	Eclectic	6	2

P = 0.344 (McNemar test, Siegel, Non-parametric Statistics).

All but one of the residents increased their Drug Knowledge Test score. This difference is significant ($t=9.22$, $df=23$, $P<0.005$). It is intriguing that the difference in knowledge between psychotherapeutic residents (mean score 79.5) and eclectic residents (mean score 87) now becomes significant, although it was not so in the beginning, as is to be observed in Table 3.

TABLE 3
Ideology Related to Amount of Psychopharmacologic Knowledge After a Six-Month Training Program

	Psychotherapeutic	Eclectic	Total
Number of residents	14	10	24
Mean score of psycho-pharmacologic knowledge	79.5*	87*	82.6

* Difference between "psychotherapeutic" and "eclectic" group is significant, $t = 1.9$, $df = 22$, $P < 0.05$.

In order to determine if there were differences in amount of knowledge about various aspects of psychopharmacology after a six-month training program by our resident groups, scores on five different aspects of psychopharmacology—side effects, classification, indications and contraindications, effectiveness and dosage, and psychosocial factors—were analyzed. The eclectic residents were superior in all aspects of psychopharmacologic knowledge at the end of six months. The differences were significant only in the instances of knowledge about "side effects" and "classification." The data in Table 4 show that the residents knew most about psychosocial aspects and least about side effects and classification.

TABLE 4
Specific Knowledge of Psychopharmacology by Two Resident Groups After a Six-Month Training Program

Different Aspect of Psychopharmacol. Knowledge	Eclectic (percent)	Psychotherapeutic (percent)	Statistical Significance (t-test)
Psychosocial	93	90	n.s.
Effect and Dosage	87	84	n.s.
Indications and Contraindications	85	81	n.s.
Side Effects	82	74	P < 0.05
Classification	80	65	P < 0.05

3. *Ideology and Drug Practice*

All the patients were studied who started on psychotropic drug therapy for more than one week by different ideologic resident groups during this six-month period. The psychotherapeutic residents started 39% of their patients on drugs; the eclectic residents, 36.3%. No statistical significance is found in the difference of frequency of prescribing drugs for inpatients between these two resident groups. It is interesting to note that ideology does not cause

TABLE 5
Percentage of Patients Started on Drugs During the Six-Month Period by Two Ideology Groups*

	Psychotherapeutic	Eclectic
Mean percent of patients started on drugs in six months	39	36.3

t = 0.4, df = 22, P > 0.1. The difference between the two groups is not significant.

* Ideology grouping here is based on the ideology at the end of six months.

much difference in the drug practice. Attention should be paid to the fact that psychotherapeutic residents, with less knowledge in psychopharmacology, prescribed as frequently as their knowledgeable eclectic counterparts.

DISCUSSION

Initially, 16 residents could be classified as psychotherapeutic and eight as eclectic. Twenty-five percent of each of these groups changed their ideology within the six-month period studied. Thus, treatment ideology does not change in a single direction. One of the influences on treatment ideology is clinical experience. The beginning residents are confronted by psychotic behavior and primitive emotions and drives in the inpatient ward. Some come to regard their psychotherapeutic skills as limited,[15] and become impressed by the patient's rapid response to somatic therapy. On the other hand, there are those who become enthusiastic over psychotherapy after learning the dynamics of the patient's pathologic defenses. Such psychiatrists are usually less concerned by speed of recovery, having faith that greater self-knowledge will prevent future relapse. It is of special interest that in this hospital, with its heavy emphasis on psychodynamics, the physician's change of attitude did not occur in any one direction, at least within six months of residency.

The effect of a six-month compulsory and systematic psychopharmacology training program is difficult to differentiate from that derived from other instructive resources such as journals, drug company literature, the *Physicians' Desk Reference,* experience with patients, and general supervision. Such differentiation can be obtained only by a control group of first-year residents in the same setting at the same time, yet not involved in the psychopharmacologic teaching program. This is not feasible in a university teaching hospital.

The finding that, at the end of six months, both resident groups know most about the psychosocial factors of drug therapy and least about side effects and classification is worthy of note. This might be related to the considerable emphasis in the course on understanding the social and psychologic aspects of drugs in the total treatment program, especially within the context of psychotherapy. The resident's own motivation and the influence of analytically oriented supervisors might also serve to explain this phenomenon. However, any psychopharmacologic training program could be strengthened by more emphasis on teaching the aspects of side effects and drug classification.

The statistically significant differences in knowledge between the two groups with respect to side effects and classification are especially noteworthy. The less knowledgeable psychotherapeutic residents gave correct answers to 74% of the side effects questionnaire, as compared to 65% of the classification questionnaire, following a six-month training course. Since knowledge of side effects is extremely important to clinical safety, and knowledge of classification is helpful to rational psychopharmacology—the effects of piperazine and aliphatic phenothiazines, major and minor tranquilizers, MAO inhibitors and dibenzazepine (tricyclic) antidepressants are all quite different—the necessity for formal supervision of drug therapy throughout the remainder of the first-year residency is indicated. Freyhan's observation that in some American hospitals, "first-year residents are often given what amounts to a free hand when it comes to drug treatment," is worthy of urgent concern.[7]

It is noteworthy that no significant difference in psychopharmacologic knowledge exists between psychotherapeutic and eclectic residents at the beginning of their training. Before entering their psychiatric careers, these residents undoubtedly had opportunities to learn about drugs during medical school and internship. We assume that their medical school experiences played some part in influencing their orientation about drugs. However, differences in ideologic orientation prior to the residency were not accompanied by statistically significant differences in knowledge about drugs. Such a difference emerges only after their assuming psychiatric responsibilities, and after their exposure to a systematic psychopharmacologic course.

Our finding that psychotherapeutic residents administer drugs as frequently as eclectic residents in the treatment of inpatients disputes any assumption that since psychotherapeutic residents administer relatively few drugs their deficiencies in drug knowledge need not be a matter of concern. It is a matter of speculation as to why no difference appears in the frequency of drug usage on the part of these two ideology groups. At least two factors suggest themselves: pressure from ward staff operative on all residents to effect immediate alleviation of psychotic behavior; also, the administration of drugs to establish a rapport for psychotherapy, a goal that might be of particular interest to the psychotherapeutically oriented residents.[24]

SUMMARY

This study was carried out at the Massachusetts Mental Health Center, a psychiatric teaching hospital of Harvard Medical School, to explore the learning of psychopharmacology by first-year residents. We were especially concerned with the influence of residents' treatment ideology on psychopharmacologic knowledge as well as practice.

Twenty-four first-year residents were studied in their first week of residency, and again after six months when the psychopharmacologic training program was finished. The results show:

1. The difference in the change of ideology between eclectic and psychotherapeutic residents in the first six months of residency is statistically not significant. The eclectic group, however, increased from 33% to 42%, whereas the psychotherapeutic group decreased from 67% to 58%.

2. Both psychotherapeutic and eclectic residents show a statistically significant increase in drug knowledge after a six-month training program. Ideology did influence learning. Though initially eclectic and psychotherapeutic residents showed no significant variance in their total amount of psychopharmacologic knowledge, after six months there was a statistically significant difference between these two groups, in favor of the eclectic residents.

3. The ideology of the first-year resident does not make significant difference in administering drugs. Psychotherapeutic residents know significantly less about side effects and classification than the eclectic residents, but they prescribe drugs for inpatients just as frequently. A special effort to teach drug treatment to the psychotherapeutic resident and to supervise his use of drugs must thus be made.

The necessity for supervision of first-year residents' drug practice is stressed.

REFERENCES

1. Azima, H., and Sarwer-Foner, G. J.: Extrapyramidal System and Neuroleptics: *Psychoanalytic Formulations of Effect on Drugs in Pharmacotherapy*, Montreal, Canada: Editions Psychiatriques, 1961, p. 507.
2. Havens, L. L.: Problems With Use of Drugs in Psychotherapy of Psychotic Patients, *Psychiatry*, 26:289–296, August 1963.
3. Ostow, M.: *Drugs in Psychoanalysis and Psychotherapy*, New York: Basic Books, 1962.
4. Semrad, E. V., and Klerman, G. L.: "Discussion of 'The Complementary Roles of Psychoanalysis and Drug Therapy' by M. Ostow," in Philip Solomon (ed.): *Psychiatric Drugs*, New York: Grune & Stratton, 1965.
5. Barton, W. E.: Training Drug Safety, *Amer. J. Psychiat.*, 121:720–721, January 1965.
6. Klerman, G. L.: Teaching of Psychopharmacology in Psychiatric Residency, *Compr. Psychiat.*, 6(4):221–226, August 1965.

7. Freyhan, F. A.: On Psychopharmacology of Psychiatric Education, *Compr. Psychiat.*, 6(4):221–226, August 1965.
8. Sheperd, M.: Psychiatric Education in the U.S. and United Kingdom: Similarities and Contrasts, *Compr. Psychiat.*, 6(4):246–254, August 1965.
9. MacIver, J., and Redlich, F. C.: Patterns of Psychiatric Practice, *Amer. J. Psychiat.*, 115:692–697, February 1959.
10. Sharaf, M. R., and Levinson, D.F.: "Patterns of Ideology and Role Definition Among Psychiatric Residents," in Greenblatt, M., Levinson, D. J., and William, R. H. (eds.): *The Patient and the Mental Hospital*, Glencoe, Ill.: Free Press, 1957, pp. 263–285.
11. Gildea, E. F.: "Teaching Psychiatry to Residents," in Arieti, Silvano (ed.): *American Handbook of Psychiatry*, New York: Basic Books, 1959, vol. 2, pp. 1935–1947.
12. Sargent, W.: Psychiatric Treatment: Here and In England, *Atlantic Monthly*, July 1964, pp. 88–95.
13. Pasamanick, B., and Rettig, S.: Status and Work Satisfaction of Psychiatrists, *Arch. Neurol. Psychiat.*, 81:399, March 1959.
14. Sharaf, M. R., and Levinson, D. J.: Quest for Omnipotence in Professional Training, *Psychiatry*, 27:135–149, May 1964.
15. Gallagher, E., Levinson, D. J., Erlick, Iza: Some Sociopsychological Characteristics of Patients and Their Relevance for Psychiatric Treatment, *Psychiatry*, 11:357–379.
16. Greenblatt, M., Levinson, D. J., and Williams, R. H.: *The Patient and the Mental Hospital*, Glencoe, Ill.: Free Press, 1957.
17. Greenblatt, M., Levinson, D. J., Klerman, G. L.: *Mental Patients in Transition*, Springfield, Ill.: Charles C. Thomas, 1962.
18. Greenblatt, M., York, R., Brown, E. L.: *From Custodial to Therapeutic Care in Mental Hospitals*, New York: Russell Sage Foundation, 1955.
19. Klerman, G. L.: "Staff Attitudes, Decision Making, and Use of Drug Therapy in Mental Hospital," in Denber, H. C. B.: *Research on Therapeutic Community*, Springfield, Ill.: Charles C. Thomas, 1959, pp. 191–214.
20. Klerman, G. L., Sharaf, M. R., Holzman, M., Levinson, D. J.: Sociopsychological Characteristics of Resident Psychiatrists and Their Use of Drug Therapy, *Amer. J. Psychiat.*, 117:111–117, August 1960.
21. Appleton, W. S.: Massive Doses of Chlorpromazine, *Arch. Gen. Psychiat.*, 9:586–592, December 1963.
22. Appleton, W. S.: Snow Phenomenon: Tranquilizing the Assaultive, *Psychiatry*, 28:88–93, February 1963.
23. Mason, A. S., and Sachs, J. M.: "Measurement of Attitude Toward Tranquilizing Drugs," in *Transactions of Chemotherapy in Psychiatry*, VA Dept. Medicine and Surgery, Washington, D.C.: 2:118–133, June 1958.
24. Klett, C. J., and Lasky, J. J.: Attitudes of Hospital Staff Members Towards Mental Illness and Chemotherapy, *Dis. Nerv. Sys.*, 23:101–105, February 1962.

CHANGING PERSPECTIVES
OF PSYCHIATRIC CARE

16

Contemporary Social Disorganization and the Rise of Scientific Psychiatry: A Discussion

by THEODORE ROTHMAN

Immanuel Kant warned us 160 years ago that the subject matter of mental diseases belonged to the philosopher, not to the physician. He inadvertently prophesied the dialectic tension of the future between scientific psychiatry and its philosophic counterpart, psychiatric sciolism. Psychology had a similar struggle for its own identity. Comte, 140 years ago, gave respectability to psychology as a science when he classified it as such, differentiating it from philosophy. The chair of psychology at universities previously had been pre-empted by philosophy. The dialectic struggles among scientific psychology, scientific psychiatry, and the philosophic approaches were live issues when this author was a student at Clark University. The history of medicine is replete with buried sciolisms that disappeared when scientific experimental methods displaced speculation. As late as our mid-century, sciolism played a significant role in psychiatry as a result of the general acceptance of the popular philosophic approaches. Phenomenology, existential philosophies, Freudian psychoanalytic ideologies, combined with theoretic sociologies, continue to play a formidable role in psychiatry. The rational guesses, speculations, and the jargon of this combined potpourri are harmonious with the McLuhanism, pop art, literature, and social and metaphysic movements of our time, which are antithetic to contemporary science and technology.

With the arrival of psychopharmacology, psychiatry was able to become unified with the current scientific methods of medicine, psychology, biology, and empiric sociology. As Magendie believed, pharmacology is based on physiologic methods, the latter effecting a closer relationship with physics and chemistry. Through psychopharmacology the gap between medicine and psychiatry closed, and psychiatry was brought closer to the basic and medical sciences.

The discovery of chlorpromazine (Thorazine) and its proven use as an antipsychotic agent, so fortuitously timed, proved most fortunate for the destiny of the scientific method in psychiatry. Because of the urgent needs of an explosive era, our society was well prepared to accept treatment with phenothiazines, tricyclic drugs, monoamine oxidase (MAO) inhibitors, and the other psychoactive agents that were relatively certain to help. The drug industry, seeking enormous profits, enthusiastically supported the scientific method of research and development in psychiatry and allied disciplines. The federal and state bureaucracies involved with public health, research, and development increased their ever pervading power by rendering full backing to scientific methods in psychiatry as well as support to interdisciplinary research, thus ensuring the safety and usefulness of the newly discovered drugs.

Simultaneously, most federal and state hospitals were bursting with an ever expanding and unmanageable population of mentally ill patients. Increasing the number of hospital beds and improving the care in these facilities had become an overwhelming administrative problem. There was no place to move the patients except into their own homes and communities. Psychoactive agents became the necessary vaccines and antibiotic drugs of the mentally ill. The widespread use of psychoactive drugs virtually made it possible to release enormous masses of patients from the overcrowded hospitals. Millions of dollars were provided by federal and state governments, and grants for applied hospital research were made by the drug industry, in an effort to prevent rehospitalization as well as first hospitalizations. Research psychiatry was warmly espoused and supported, though all too many of the research programs were hurriedly devised and promoted. The universities, the psychiatric and psychologic associations, failed to play a primary role in these overwhelming developments except for publishing a profusion of papers blueprinting theoretic formulations for community and social psychiatry. What remains most significant was that during the transition the scientific method was being widely applied in psychiatry, and that empiric sociology proved itself a valuable ally in providing a solid base for the pragmatic changes.

Moral philosophers, like Montaigne, and the Greco-Roman and Judaic-Christian ethics originated the historic roots of moral therapy. Pinel, Tuke, and Conolly, who popularized moral therapy for the mentally ill, became our contemporaries. The moral therapy for the mentally ill was of course an ancient tradition in psychiatry and was generally practiced by the better hospitals and psychiatrists. With the social and political changes during the 19th century due to the industrial revolution, problems of immigration, overpopulation, and urbanization followed. Moral therapy fell into temporary disuse.

Recent approaches, such as the therapeutic community, short hospitalization, community care, and the reintegration and rehabilitation of the mentally ill, are indeed revived versions of moral therapy—rediscovered to fit the welfare state programs of a changing political and social democracy. Moral therapy harmonized with the ideologies of the administrative bureaucracy of federal and state governments, which, following Parkinson's Law, needed to expand new programs. The public health approaches encouraged scientific psychiatry to utilize the methods of preventive medicine and seek out the biostatistic services for a new epidemiology, ecology, and empiric sociology of the mentally ill. Biostatistics, programming, and computers became necessary tools in psychiatry to investigate clinical trials, to compare therapies, and to make future projections of population trends of the mentally ill. Psychiatry to a large extent became dependent on the approval of federal and state granting agencies. The federal government therefore frequently set the tone and goals of scientific psychiatry.

This then is the turbulent atmosphere and historic period in which this volume was written and compiled. The contributors are research scientists, competent investigators interested in promoting better scientific approaches. Our book has described their roots in the past and in the present, thus offering living illustrations of some of the new work being accomplished in scientific psychiatry. The application of the biostatistic services and empiric sociology is present in most of the chapters. The manner in which psychopharmacology has helped evolve a more scientific psychiatry in the treatment of schizophrenia and affective disorders is reflected throughout this book. The manner in which the basic therapeutic patterns have changed and the cultural lag in teaching these changes are quite thoroughly covered. The discarding of the jargon of sciolism is evident. Throughout this volume there is firm emphasis on the fact that a few subtypes of patients may benefit by treatments that differ from those usually considered beneficial to a statistically significant number of patients.

What *Changing Patterns in Psychiatric Care* would seem to prove is that scientific psychiatry definitely benefits the mentally ill; that moral therapy is a living conceptual framework that can be widely used in the mental health services harmonizing with our present political and social programs; that any surviving sciolisms of the past tend only to blur psychiatry's main goals. Our purpose is to label philosophic approaches as rational speculation or as occasional irrational guessing. Open-mindedness is our keynote—in clinical treatment, in research, and in educational approaches. Humility is encouraged by the new and evolving science.

Today's advances augur well for psychiatry as a medical science —we can expect medicine and medical education to be further enriched with many new contributions. The chapters comprising this volume are specific illustrations of only a few of the changing patterns of psychiatric care that merit replication by other psychiatrists.

But beware! There is always a philosophic, social, or political movement lurking around the corner that could divert psychiatry to some new-sounding sciolism. Observe the recent efflorescence of political action groups, T-groups, the infinite number of group psychotherapies, the sensitivity training programs, and the gestalt and nude therapies. O shades of Mesmer! Man has never completely ceased his search for instant magic!

Index

Ackerknecht, E. H., 19
Ackner, B., 23, 23 t
ACNP. *See* American College of Neuropsychopharmacology
Action for Mental Health (Joint Commission on Mental Illness and Health), 32
Adler, Alfred, 16, 18
Agitation-excitement, 78 fig., 80
Akathisia, 167 t, 169, 177, 182
Alcoholism, 63, 78 fig., 79, 80, 81
Alexander, F., 18
Allen, M., 13
Alpha-methyl-dopa
  effect of, on brain amines, 217 t, 220
Alvig, 206
American College of Neuropsychopharmacology (ACNP), xv, xxi
American Handbook of Psychiatry, 268
American Psychiatric Association, 235
American Psychoanalytic Association
  Central Fact Finding Committee Report of, 15 t, 17, 18
Amitriptyline HCl (Elavil), 28, 54, 97, 200, 201
  effectiveness of, compared with ETC, 208
  inpatient use of, 48 t, 49, 50, 51 t, 52
  response of VA patients to, measured by IMPS, 205 t
Amitriptyline (HCl) and perphenazine, combined
  response of VA patients to, measured by IMPS, 205 t
Amobarbital, 54
Amobarbital and dextroamphetamine, combined
  response of VA patients to, measured by IMPS, 205 t
Amphetamine, 198
  and other psychomotor stimulants, 203–204
  effect of, on brain amines, 222
  studies of, 222
Amphetamine and chlorpromazine, combined, 204
"Analysis Terminable and Interminable" (Freud), 17
Andreani, 212 t
Anhedonia, 127, 209
Antidepressant therapies and drugs
  effects of, on brain levels of NE and serotonin, 217 t, 218, 219–24
Antidepressants, 6, 85
  amphetamine and other psychomotor stimulants, 203–204
  combination therapy, 204–206
  compared with ECT, 207–208
  inpatient use of, 48 t, 48–49, 50, 51 t, 52
  monoamine oxidase (MAO) inhibitors, 28, 197, 198, 201–203. *See also* Monoamine oxidase inhibitors
  phenothiazines, 204–206. *See also* Phenothiazines
  results of treatment of VA patients classified by Overall-Hollister subtypes, by type of drug, 204, 205 t

Antidepressants (*Cont.*)
  tricyclic, 28, 197, 198–201. *See also* Tricyclic antidepressants
  use of, by general practitioner, 54
Antiparkinson drugs, 167 t
  use of, with depot fluphenazines, 177–78, 180, 181, 182, 183
Anxiety-depression, 78 fig., 80, 84–85
Anxious intropunitiveness, measurement of, 154, 163 t
Apathy and retardation, measurement of 154, 163 t, 164
Appearance or behavior, inappropriate or bizarre, 78 fig., 79, 80
Appleby, L., 261
Appleton, William S., 56–57, 267–78
Arlidge, J. T., 13
Ashburner, 212 t
Ataractic agents, 28
  value of, in prevention of hospitalization of schizophrenic outpatients, 109–15
Atropine
  response of VA patients to, measured by IMPS, 205 t
Austin, H., 124 n
Aventyl. *See* Nortriptyline HCl
Awl, William M., 19
Ayd, F., 190

Baastrup, P. C., 211, 212 t, 212–13
Baker, Cecil G., 149 n
Barbiturates, 21, 54
Beers, Clifford, 31
Behavior or appearance, inappropriate or bizarre, 78 fig., 79, 80
Behavior therapy, 15 t, 19
Belladonna, 21
Bellevue Hospital, 72, 73, 82–84, 86–87, 88
Belligerence-hostile, measurement of, 153, 154, 160, 162 t, 163 t
Belligerence-negativism, 78 fig., 80, 81
Belling, 212 t
Benactyzine HCl and Meprobamate (Deprol)
  inpatient use of, 48 t, 49, 51 t
  outpatient use of, 206
Berg, K., 101
Bernheim, H., 14–15, 15 t
Bethlem Hospital, 7, 8
  results of treatment in, 8, 8 t
Binet, Alfred, xix
Bini, L., 24
Binner, P. R., 33
Binstock, William A., 96
Biogenic amine hypothesis, 216–25
  outline of factors in, 217 t
Bird, E. G., 27
Bleuler, Paul, xix, 13, 236, 239
Bloomingdale Asylum, results of psychiatric treatment in, 8 t, 11
Bockoven, J. S., 11
Bonato, Roland R., 149 n
Bond, E. D., 22, 23, 23 t, 24
Borsa, J. A., 27

285